ANESTHESIA AND ANALGESIA IN DERMATOLOGIC SURGERY

T0173820

BASIC AND CLINICAL DERMATOLOGY

Series Editors

Alan R. Shalita, M.D.
Distinguished Teaching Professor and Chairman
Department of Dermatology
SUNY Downstate Medical Center
Brooklyn, New York

David A. Norris, M.D.
Director of Research
Professor of Dermatology
The University of Colorado
Health Sciences Center
Denver, Colorado

ANESTHESIA AND ANALGESIA IN DERMATOLOGIC SURGERY

Edited by

Marwali Harahap
University of North Sumatra
Medan, Indonesia

Adel R. Abadir
Brookdale University Hospital
Brooklyn, New York, USA

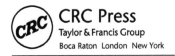

CRC Press
Taylor & Francis Group
Boca Raton   London   New York

CRC Press is an imprint of the
Taylor & Francis Group, an **informa** business

First published 2008 by Informa Healthcare USA, Inc.

Published 2018 by CRC Press
Taylor & Francis Group
6000 Broken Sound Parkway NW, Suite 300
Boca Raton, FL 33487-2742

© 2008 by Taylor & Francis Group, LLC
CRC Press is an imprint of Taylor & Francis Group, an Informa business

First issued in paperback 2019

No claim to original U.S. Government works

ISBN 13: 978-0-367-45273-5 (pbk)
ISBN 13: 978-0-8493-3698-0 (hbk)

**Visit the Taylor & Francis Web site at
http://www.taylorandfrancis.com**

**and the CRC Press Web site at
http://www.crcpress.com**

Library of Congress Cataloging-in-Publication Data

Anesthesia and analgesia in dermatologic surgery / edited by Marwali Harahap, Adel R. Abadir.
    p. ; cm. — (Basic and clinical dermatology ; 42)
    Includes bibliographical references and index.
    ISBN-13: 978-0-8493-3698-0 (hardcover : alk. paper)
    ISBN-10: 0-8493-3698-8 (hardcover : alk. paper)
    1. Anesthesia. 2. Analgesia. 3. Skin—Surgery. I. Harahap, Marwali.
II. Abadir, Adel R. III. Series.
    [DNLM: 1. Analgesia—methods—Handbooks.
2. Anesthesia—methods—Handbooks. 3. Dermatology—methods—Handbooks.
4. Skin—surgery—Handbooks. 5. Skin Diseases—surgery—Handbooks. W1
CL69L v.42 2008 / WO 231 A5322 2008]
  RD82.A6593 2008
  617.9′6—dc22
                        2007043379

Series Introduction

In the past 30 years, there has been a vast explosion in new information relating to the art and science of dermatology as well as fundamental cutaneous biology. Furthermore, this information is no longer of interest only to the small but growing specialty of dermatology. Clinicians and scientists from a wide variety of disciplines have come to recognize both the importance of skin in fundamental biological processes and the broad implications of understanding the pathogenesis of skin disease. As a result, there is now a multidisciplinary and worldwide interest in the progress of dermatology.

With these factors in mind, we have undertaken this series of books specifically oriented to dermatology. The scope of the series is purposely broad, with books ranging from pure basic science to practical, applied clinical dermatology. Thus, while there is something for everyone, all volumes in the series will ultimately prove to be valuable additions to the dermatologist's library.

Anesthesia and pain management have long been treated as a secondary issue in dermatology and dermatological surgery. This volume, by leading practitioners in the field, not only demonstrates the importance of understanding the proper use of these modalities, but is also a practical guide for the clinician.

Alan R. Shalita, M.D.
SUNY Downstate Medical Center
Brooklyn, New York, U.S.A.

Preface

Anesthesia and analgesia are exceptionally important therapeutic tools. Their preeminence in pain control for dermatologic surgery is underscored by their widespread use. Without availability of anesthesia and analgesia, much of dermatologic surgery considered routine today would be difficult or impossible to perform.

This book is designed for practitioners of dermatologic surgery who use anesthesia and analgesia on a daily basis throughout their professional careers. It may also be of interest to certain physicians, who are called upon to administer anesthesia and analgesia for skin problems.

Dermatologists have always been at the forefront of new developments for treating the skin and doing so in the least painful fashion. We do so many procedures each day on fully awake patients with minimal discomfort.

The text has been prepared to be comprehensive, providing the basic concepts needed to fully understand the drugs and techniques and how they work, with step-by-step descriptions of the various techniques. Until very recently, a book dealing with the combined subjects of anesthesia and analgesia for dermatologic surgery was not available. The purpose of producing such a volume is to make available concentrated information on particular aspects of these subjects.

In this book we have attempted to draw together the current state of knowledge on all aspects of topical anesthesia. In the past, most topical anesthetics were only able to penetrate mucosal surfaces. With the development of the eutectic mixture that penetrates through intact skin, we have been able to provide effective analgesia for a wide range of superficial surgical procedures, including the harvesting of split skin grafts, laser surgery, electrosurgery, epilation, and skin biopsy.

The basic principles of regional and local anesthesia are discussed with respect to anatomy, local anesthetic agent, and techniques. With nerve blocks we can achieve large areas of anesthesia with few injections. When done correctly, regional nerve blocks obviate the need for excessive sedation or general anesthesia. The goal is to organize an approach to regional blocks with clear anatomic landmarks that will assist the surgeon in achieving complete facial analgesia. These nerve blocks can be used before many of our procedures, such as chemical peels, laser surgery, and large reconstruction. Mastery of regional anesthesia can serve us well.

Tumescent anesthesia, the subcutaneous infiltration of a large volume of very dilute lidocaine and epinephrine that causes the targeted tissue to become swollen and firm or tumescent, is also discussed. The development of the tumescent technique, with its use in eliminating the problems of blood loss, fluid shifts, and general anesthesia, will drastically change the approach to this popular procedure.

The contributors, acknowledged authorities in their respective fields, explore a variety of important issues in anesthesia and analgesia for dermatologic surgery, including local anesthesia and anesthetic solutions, vasoconstrictors, patient evaluation and choice of anesthetics as well as conscious sedation and a look at potential complications and emergencies that might arise. A chapter focusing on pediatric patients outlines the special problems that need to be addressed for this patient population. A variety of sedative and hypnotic agents may be used for pediatric dermatology procedures, and guidelines for their appropriate use have been published.

In this book, a chapter on iontophoresis has been included, which discusses future developments in pain control in dermatologic surgery. It allows us to use every option from electricity to various medicines including lidocaine into the skin. Its usefulness is expanding, and its applications are sure to increase in the years to come.

Another chapter describes a valuable new technique for dermatologic surgery. Nitrous oxide–oxygen is effective and probably safer than presently used agents for abating pain and anxiety. It has not been widely employed in the practice of dermatologic surgery. The dental surgeons' many years of experience with this technique suggests that it could be useful as an adjunct to anesthesia and analgesia in dermatologic surgery. Nitrous oxide is an excellent agent for the pre–anesthetic induction phase of hair transplantation surgery. It is of great help in reducing pain from local anesthetic infiltration and has an extremely low complication profile. Except for hair transplantation surgery, it may prove to be a valuable agent in other dermatologic surgery procedures, such as chemical peeling, liposuction, and skin cancer surgery.

Commensurate with the demands of increasing levels of sophistication of dermatologic surgery, an established anesthesia technique called conscious sedation has been employed. Conscious sedation has been defined as a medically controlled state of depressed consciousness that allows protective reflexes to be maintained, retains the patient's ability to maintain a patent airway continuously, and permits appropriate responses by the patient to physical stimulation or verbal command. Conscious sedation is appropriate for outpatient ambulatory surgical procedures. However, it should be emphasized that office use is contingent on suitable office settings and administration by trained individuals.

The dermatologic surgeon should be keenly aware of the possibility of postoperative pain and of the particular procedures that are most likely to cause it. The discomforts of postoperative pain are best alleviated by either analgetics or narcotics. Not all patients require narcotics, since the less potent analgetics often eliminate the patients' discomfort very well.

We hope that the work gathered will prove useful to all health care professionals involved in the care of patients undergoing dermatologic surgery.

Contents

Contributors

Christie T. Ammirati   Department of Dermatology, Penn State Milton S. Hershey Medical Center, Hershey, Pennsylvania, U.S.A.

Emil Bisaccia   Department of Dermatology, Columbia University, New York, New York, U.S.A.

Eckart Haneke   Department of Dermatology Clinic, Freiburg, Germany; Department of Dermatology, Inselspital, University of Berne, Berne, Switzerland; and Department of Dermatology, Academic Hospital, University of Ghent, Ghent, Belgium

William B. Henghold   The Skin Cancer Center of NW Florida, Pensacola, Florida, U.S.A.

George J. Hruza   Laser and Dermatologic Surgery Center, Town and Country and Department of Dermatology and Otolaryngology/Head and Neck Surgery, St. Louis University School of Medicine, St. Louis, Missouri, U.S.A.

Conway C. Huang   Department of Dermatology, University of Alabama at Birmingham, Birmingham, Alabama, U.S.A.

Paul O. Larson   Retired, Mohs Surgery Clinic, University of Wisconsin, Madison, Wisconsin, U.S.A.

Brent R. Moody   Vanderbilt University Medical Center, Nashville, Tennessee, U.S.A.

Thierry Pirotte   Department of Anesthesiology, Cliniques Universitaires Saint-Luc, Brussels, Belgium

D. Roseeuw   Department of Dermatology, University Hospital Brussels (UZ Brussel), Brussels, Belgium

Neil S. Sadick   Department of Dermatology, Joan and Sanford I. Weill Medical College and Weill Cornell Graduate School of Medical Sciences, Cornell University, New York, New York, U.S.A.

Dwight Scarborough   Cosmetic Surgery Center, Ohio State University, Dublin, Ohio, U.S.A.

S. 't Kint   Department of Dermatology, University Hospital Brussels (UZ Brussel), Brussels, Belgium

Omar Torres   Cosmetic Surgery and Dermatology, PLLC, St. Luke's-Roosevelt Medical Center, Department of Dermatology, Columbia University, New York, New York, U.S.A.

Francis Veyckemans   Department of Anesthesiology, Cliniques Universitaires Saint-Luc, Brussels, Belgium

William T. Zempsky   Connecticut Children's Medical Center and University of Connecticut School of Medicine, Hartford, Connecticut, U.S.A.

1

Local Anesthetics and Anesthetic Solutions: Classification, Mode of Action and Dosages

Eckart Haneke

*Department of Dermatology Clinic,
Freiburg, Germany;
Department of Dermatology, Inselspital,
University of Berne, Berne, Switzerland; and
Department of Dermatology, Academic Hospital,
University of Ghent, Ghent, Belgium*

INTRODUCTION

Local anesthetics have revolutionized surgery and many more medical subspecialties. The first local anesthetic ever used was cocaine, which remained for many years the only active substance and also the standard until procaine was synthesized.

Local anesthetics are used for surface (topical), infiltration, regional and plexus blocks, epidural, and intrathecal anesthesias. The aim of local anesthesia is to make the skin and mucous membranes, as well as deeper tissues, insensitive to pain. Blockade of sensory and motoric functions depends on the concentration and amount of the local anesthetic used.

Local anesthetics impair the generation and transmission of nerve impulses. They act both on all types of nerve cells as well as the peripheral nervous tissue, on efferent motor, and on autonomous as well as afferent sensory nerves. The action on smooth and striated muscles as well as sweat glands is inhibited depending on the action on their innervating nerves.

The effect of all local anesthetics is time dependent, and nerve function is fully restored after a certain period of time depending on the action profile of the drug. Generally, sensory functions are blocked for a longer period than motor ones.

MECHANISM OF ACTION

Local anesthetics block both the initiation and conduction of nerve impulses by decreasing the neuronal membrane's permeability to sodium ions, perhaps by attaching to a site on the sodium channel. This reversibly stabilizes the membrane and inhibits depolarization, resulting in the failure of a propagated action potential and subsequent conduction blockade.

The concentration of drug needed to block large nerve trunks is greater than that needed for smaller peripheral nerves.

The depth of anesthesia depends on the degree by which nerve fibers are myelinated and ensheathed by Schwann cells, and from the local anesthetic's water and lipid solubility at the given local tissue pH. Thin nerve fibers are more easily blocked than thick ones. However, once the local anesthetic has reached its target, myelinated fibers are more readily blocked than unmyelinated ones because of the need to produce blockade only at the nodes of Ranvier. In general, autonomic (B and C fibers), small unmyelinated (C fibers), and small myelinated fibers (B and Aδ fibers) will be more readily blocked than thick, myelinated fibers (Aα and Aβ fibers). Thus, a differential block can be achieved where the smaller pain and autonomic fibers are blocked, while larger touch and motor fibers are spared. This difference is due to the fact that nerve fibers containing myelin are relatively impervious to local anesthetic solutions compared to those that contain little or no myelin.

Local anesthetics are weakly alkaline and are kept in solution as salts. In order to become active, the drug has to be transformed into a lipophilic substance that can penetrate the nerve cells. Intracellularly, the base is dissociated again and becomes active. In the slightly acidic milieu of an inflamed tissue, the anesthetic is mainly dissociated and its penetration into the nerve cell is more difficult, resulting in decreased activity.

Local anesthetics in solution exist in a chemical equilibrium between the basic uncharged form (B) and the charged cationic form (BH$^+$). At a certain hydrogen concentration specific for each drug, the concentration of the local anesthetic base is equal to that of the charged cation. This hydrogen concentration is called the pK_a. This relationship is expressed as

$$pH = pK_a + \left(\frac{B}{BH^+} \right)$$

A lower pK_a means that a greater fraction of the molecules exists in the unionized form in the body, so they more easily cross nerve membranes leading to faster onset. The pK_a of currently used local anesthetic compounds lies between 7.7 and 8.5. The commercially available solutions are always acidic, so that they contain more ionized molecules. Acidosis in the environment into which the local anesthetic is injected (as is present in an infected or inflamed tissue) further increases the ionized fraction of drugs. This is consistent with slower onset and poor quality of local anesthesia when a local anesthetic is injected into an acidic infected area. The lipid solubility and pK_a of the local anesthetic are the primary determinants of the degree of differential blockade.

There is complete systemic absorption for all injected local anesthetics. The rate of absorption is influenced by the site and route of administration (especially the vascularity or rate of blood flow at the injection site), the total dose (volume and concentration) administered, physical characteristics (such as degree of protein binding and lipid solubility) of the individual agent, and whether or not a vasoconstrictor is used concurrently.

TYPES OF LOCAL ANESTHETICS

The new synthetic local anesthetics were developed in early 1900, after cocaine had been in use for more than 20 years. The chemical structure of most synthetic anesthetics comprises a benzene ring and a short aliphatic chain with a secondary or tertiary amine. These are bound together either by an ester or amide bond. The two groups are different in their metabolism, chemical stability, and allergenicity. Esters are rapidly inactivated by hydrolytic enzymes in the blood plasma. The amide-type local anesthetics are metabolized in the liver by amidases.

The degree to which local anesthetic substances have systemic effects depends on their rate of metabolic breakdown and of uptake into the bloodstream. This balance varies from substance to substance, but also from person to person, for the same substance. Some of those local anesthetics with an unfavorable profile are therefore only used on the skin surface.

Nowadays, the most important local anesthetics are those of the amide type. There are now many substances available, but the most widely used in dermatologic surgery are

- Lidocaine
- Mepivacaine
- Prilocaine
- Bupivacaine and its levo-enantiomer levo-bupivacaine
- Ropivacaine
- Articaine

As mentioned above, their anesthetic properties differ, but may considerably vary from the values given below, depending on the injection site, the mode of anesthesia (infiltration, block, intrathecal, etc.), addition of vasoconstrictors or buffers, and tissue pH (Table 1).

Table 1   Properties of the Most Commonly Used Local Anesthetics

Anesthetic compound	Time needed to become active (min)	Anesthetic period	Type of anesthetic
Lidocaine[a]	5	30 min–1 hr	Amide
Mepivacaine[a]	4	1–3 hr	Amide
Prilocaine[a]	3	2–2.5 hr	Amide
Bupivacain[a]	8	3–7 hr	Amide
Ropivacaine[a]	1–15	30 min–6 hr	Amide
Articaine[a]	5	1–3 hr	Amide

[a]Considerably higher doses are used for tumescence local anesthesia.

Procaine and other ester-type local anesthetics are much less used because of their relatively short action period and the risk of allergic side effects.

Inactivation

Ester-type local anesthetics are inactivated by plasma esterases, and amide-type ones have a mostly hepatic metabolism. However, articaine is an amide-type local anesthetic with an ester bond and is inactivated by plasma esterases.

Elimination

Excretion is via the kidneys, primarily as metabolites. For some of these agents, including lidocaine, mepivacaine, and tetracaine, renal excretion may follow biliary excretion into, and reabsorption from, the gastrointestinal tract.

The quantity of dose excreted unchanged is as follows: articaine 2–5%, bupivacaine 5%, etidocaine < 10%, lidocaine 10%, levobupivacaine 0%, mepivacaine 5–10%, procaine < 2%.

Allergy Risk

Patients allergic to para-aminobenzoic acid (PABA) or parabens may be sensitive to procaine, chloroprocaine, or tetracaine also. They may also be sensitive to other local anesthetic solutions containing parabens as preservatives.

There is a high cross-allergy risk among all the ester-type anesthetics.

True allergies to amide-type local anesthetics are very rare, and infrequently the patients may be sensitive to other amide-type local anesthetics.

Cross-sensitivity between ester-type local anesthetics and amide-type local anesthetics has not been described, though one may have two independent allergies.

Local Anesthetics in Pregnancy

Local anesthetics cross the placenta depending on their binding to plasma proteins. Only the free substance will reach the fetal circulation. The blood volume increases during pregnancy, mainly because of an increase of the plasma volume, thus decreasing the concentration of plasma proteins. The biologically active drug concentration rises. Substances such as articaine, bupivacaine, or etidocaine, which have a plasma protein binding of over 90%, are therefore preferable to lidocaine, mepivacaine, or prilocaine, with a plasma protein binding of less than 70%. Also, the more lipophilic a substance, the more it crosses the placenta (1–4).

GENERAL ADVERSE SIDE EFFECTS

Most side effects of local anesthetics are due to overdosing or intravasal injection. Commonly, they appear as signs of disturbances of organ systems in which nerve conduction plays an important role, such as the central nervous and the cardiovascular systems. Which adverse effect develops is dependent on the rate of diffusion of the anesthetic into the blood circulation. In case of rapid penetration from the tissue into the bloodstream, anxiousness, confusion, speech troubles, visual and acoustic disturbances, later muscle contraction, so-called twitches, and also hypertension and tachycardia may develop. In case of intravasal injection, tremor and muscle cramps may appear directly. With increasing blood levels, convulsions, apnea due to inhibition of the respiratory center and cardiac arrest due to blockade of myocardial stimulation, and stimulus transmission develop. The latter are mainly seen in slowly metabolized amide-type anesthetics such as bupivacaine, but may also develop in liver disease where the metabolic breakdown of lidocaine and other amides is considerably decreased. Furthermore, both metabolic and respiratory acidosis as well as heart, liver, and kidney diseases may slow down the metabolism of amide-type local anesthetics. Systemic toxicity may be more likely to occur in geriatric patients.

An adverse effect unique to prilocaine is methemoglobinemia.

Another type of adverse effect may be related to the specific site, with or without the addition of a vasoconstrictor; the best-known is the temporary or permanent loss of vision after accidental intravasal injection into the angular artery, which can lead to fluid emboli that occlude the central retinal artery.

In contrast, hypersensitivity reactions are almost exclusively seen in ester-type local anesthetics because of the generation of PABA, which develops through hydrolysis of the substance. These reactions are not foreseeable. They are characterized by a macular to urticarial rash, bronchospasm, angioedema, even anaphylactic shock with fatal outcome.

Lasting numbness after local anesthesia, particularly after a digital block, is not due to the local anesthetic substance but to nerve injury from the cutting tip of the injection needle.

INTERACTIONS

A large number of drugs may interfere with local anesthetics, although to a variable degree. In these cases, the physician may have to change the dose, or other precautions may be necessary. A drug history is therefore mandatory.

- β-Adrenergic blocking agents [carteolol, e.g., Cartrol; carvedilol, e.g., Coreg; labetolol, e.g., Normodyne; nadolol, e.g., Corgard; oxprenolol, e.g., Trasicor; penbutolol, e.g., Levatol; pindolol, e.g., Visken; propranolol, e.g., Inderal; sotalol, e.g., Sotacor; timolol, e.g., Blocadren; or Carteolol (ophthalmic), e.g., Ocupress; Levobunolol (ophthalmic), e.g., Betagan; Metipranolol (ophthalmic), e.g., OptiPranolol; or Timolol (ophthalmic), e.g., Timoptic.]

Use of some local anesthetics with these medicines may increase the risk of high blood pressure or a slow heart rate.

- Central nervous system (CNS) depressants (medicines that cause drowsiness)

Use of local anesthetics with these medicines may increase the risk of drowsiness.

- Digoxin (e.g., Lanoxin)

Use of some local anesthetics with digoxin may increase the risk of irregular heartbeats.

- Haloperidol (e.g., Haldol) or phenothiazines (e.g., Phenergan)

Use of these neuroleptics may reduce the effectiveness of the local anesthetic.

- Tricyclic antidepressants (amitriptyline, e.g., Elavil; amoxapine, e.g., Asendin; clomipramine, e.g., Anafranil; desipramine, e.g., Norpramin; doxepin, e.g., Sinequan; imipramine, e.g., Tofranil; nortriptyline, e.g., Aventyl; protriptyline, e.g., Vivactil; trimipramine, e.g., Surmontil; or maprotiline, e.g., Ludiomil)

Use of some local anesthetics may increase the chance of high blood pressure and irregular heartbeats.

- Any other medicine, prescription or nonprescription [over-the-counter (OTC)], or "street" drugs, such as amphetamines ("uppers"), barbiturates ("downers"), cocaine (including "crack"), marijuana, phencyclidine (PCP, "angel dust"), and heroin or other narcotics

Serious side effects may occur if anyone gets a local anesthetic without the physician's knowing that another medicine is being taken.

OTHER MEDICAL PROBLEMS

The presence of other medical problems may affect the use of local anesthetics. The physician should ask for any other medical problems, especially

- Asthma
  Increased chance of allergic-like reactions with use of some local anesthetics
- Brain infection or tumor or blood clotting disorders
  Increased chance of bleeding with injection of local anesthetics
- Diabetes mellitus
  Use of local anesthetics can cause stress on the heart in case of diabetes mellitus.
- Heart disease
  Use of local anesthetics can worsen some kinds of heart disease.
- History of migraine headaches
  Use of local anesthetics can worsen headaches.
- Hypertension (high blood pressure) or hypotension (low blood pressure)
  Use of local anesthetics can cause hypotension or hypertension.
- Hyperthyroidism
  Use of local anesthetics can cause stress on the heart in case of hyperthyroidism.
- Kidney disease or liver disease
  Use of some local anesthetics can increase the chances of side effects.
- Methemoglobinemia
  Prilocaine may exacerbate methemoglobinemia.
- Peripheral vascular disease
  Use of some local anesthetics can exacerbate peripheral vascular disease or increase blood pressure.
- Skin infection or inflammation
  It is generally not recommended to inject a local anesthetic into infected skin.

GENERAL USE OF LOCAL ANESTHETICS

Topical anesthetics are a help for venipuncture, vaccinations, some very superficial procedures, such as curettage, shave excisions, and laser treatments, and a variety of other procedures. For small- and medium-sized dermatologic operations, *infiltration anesthesia* is the most feasible and is performed hundreds of thousands of times daily all over the world with almost no complications. *Nerve blocks* are performed for finger and toe operations, often in the midface, more rarely by dermatologists for hand and foot surgery. A relatively new technique is the *transthecal anesthesia* for fingernail surgery. *Peridural anesthesias* are performed by anesthesiologists and are useful for the legs. *Special nerve blocks* are sometimes performed by dermatologists for particular chronic pain syndromes. The development of *tumescence anesthesia* opened new horizons for the dermatologic surgeon. Originally used for liposuction surgery, it is now widely used for many operations that formerly required general anesthesia just because of the size of the area to be anesthetized.

Accepted, though not exclusive, indications for different local anesthetics are:

Topical anesthesia—Lidocaine, lidocaine-prilocaine, lidocaine-tetracaine, and chloroprocaine are indicated.

Local infiltration—Bupivacaine (with or without epinephrine), chloroprocaine, etidocaine (with or without epinephrine), levobupivacaine, lidocaine (with or without epinephrine), mepivacaine, procaine, and ropivacaine are indicated.

Peripheral nerve block—Bupivacaine (with or without epinephrine), chloroprocaine, etidocaine (with or without epinephrine), levobupivacaine, lidocaine (with or without epinephrine), mepivacaine, procaine, and ropivacaine are indicated.

Dental infiltration or nerve block—Articaine with epinephrine, bupivacaine and epinephrine, chloroprocaine (with or without added epinephrine), etidocaine and epinephrine, lidocaine (with or without epinephrine), mepivacaine (with or without levonordefrin), and prilocaine (with or without epinephrine) are indicated. Unless specifically contraindicated, a vasoconstrictor-containing solution is preferred. However, particularly in recent time, articaine became more and more widely used for other indications such as infiltration and tumescent anesthesia.

Intravenous regional anesthesia (Bier block)—Chloroprocaine, lidocaine, and mepivacaine are indicated.

TOPICAL ANESTHETICS

There are a large number of substances with topical anesthetic properties. Many of them are not used for surgery, but more to relieve itch. Benzocaine is used for itching dermatoses as is cinchocaine. Polidocanol, an agent also used for sclerotherapy of veins and hemorrhoids, is added to certain lotions and bath oil for the treatment of atopic eczema and pruritus. Allergic reactions have often been observed with benzocaine, less frequently with cinchocaine.

These substances will be summarized together with some infrequently used anesthetics for infiltration in Table 2.

Cocaine (methyl (–) 3β-benzoyloxy-tropane-2 β-carboxylate) was isolated almost 150 years ago from the South-American bush *Erythroxylon coca* by Niemann. He noted that an extract from the leaves of this bush caused numbness of the tongue (5). In 1880, local anesthesia was produced with cocaine after subcutaneous injection (6). Only a few years later, it was used for topical ophthalmic anesthesia and for a peripheral nerve block. Cocaine continued to be the

Table 2 Topically Active Anesthetic Substances and Some Rarely Used Drugs for Infiltration Anesthesia

Amyleine (dimethylaminomethyl)-1-methyl-1-propyl benzoate

Amyleine (amylocaine) chlorhydrate

Benzocaine (4-ethyl aminobenzoate)

Benzyl alcohol (phenyl methanol)

Betoxycaine (2-(diethyl amino ethoxy)-3-amino-4-butoxy benzoate)

Betoxycaine chlorhydrate

Butacaine (3-(dibutylamino)-1-propanol 4-aminobenzoate)

Butacaine sulfate

Butoform (4-butyl aminobenzoate)

Chlorobutanol (1,1,1-trichloro-2-methyl-2-propanol)

Cinchocaine

Clemizole undecylate (4-chlorobenzyl)-1-(1-methylpyrrolidinyl)-2 benzimidazole undeceneoate.

Cocaine (methyl (–) 3β-benzoyloxytropane-2 β-carboxylate)

Cryofluorane (1,2-dichlor-1,1,2,2-tetrafluoro ethane)

Dextrocaine hydrochloride Methyl-((+)-3β-benzyloxy tropane 2α carboxylate)

Lidocaine (2-(diethylamino)-N-(2,6-dimethylphenyl) acetamide

Lidocaine hydrochloride

Myrtecaine (nopoxamine) (2-(N,N-diethyl-2-[6,6-dimethyl-2-norpinene-2 yl]-2 ethoxy)-ethylamine)

Myrtecaine laurylsulfate

Oxetacaine (N-(2-hydroxyethyl)imino-2,2-bis-(N-α,α'dimethyl N-methyl acetamide)

Oxybuprocaine hydrochloride (2-diethylaminoethyl-4-amino-3-butoxy benzoate)

Parethoxycaine hydrochloride (2-(diethyl amino)ethyl-4-ethoxy benzoate hydrochloride)

Pramocaine (4-[3-(4-butoxy phenoxy) propyl]morpholine)

Prilocaine hydrochloride (α-propylamino-2-methylpropionanilide hydrochloride)

Propanocaine (3-diéthylamino-1-phénylpropyle benzoate)

Proxymetacaine (2-(diethylamino)ethyl-3-amino-4-propoxybenzoate)

Proxymetacaine hydrochloride

Quinisocaine hydrochloride (3-butyl-1-[2-(dimethylamino)ethoxy] isoquinoleine hydrochloride)

Tetracaine (2-(dimethylamino)ethyl-4-(butylamino)benzoate)

Tetracaine hydrochloride

Tolycaine (2-(2-diethyl aminoacetamido)-m-toluate hydrochloride)

Trimebutine (2-(dimethylamino)-2-phenylbutyl-3,4,5-trimethoxybenzoate)

Trimebutine hydrochloride

only local anesthetic drug for almost a quarter century. It is still used in oph-thalmology and also in rhinoplasty surgery as a topical anesthetic agent with a long action. One major advantage is its inherent vasocontrictor action due to potentiation of the endogenous norepinephrine action of sympathetic nerve endings. The priapism observed in drug addicts after intracavernous injection is probably due to the potentiation of endogenous α-adrenergic substances.

Because of its addiction potential, its medical use is now highly restricted. Surprisingly, cocaine is still widely used as a topical anesthetic, particular in rhinoplasties. It is added as an adjunct to conventional local anesthesia by inserting cocaine solution-soaked cotton swabs into the nose. This gives excel-lent mucosal anesthesia with ischemia and makes the patient much less anxious.

Tetracaine (amethocaine) (2-(dimethylamino)-ethyl-4-(butylamino)ben-zoate) has been used in ophthalmology for approximately half a century. Der-matologists who perform laser surgery near the eye and apply eye shields also often use tetracaine drops to make the conjunctiva insensitive to the otherwise uncomfortable procedure of inserting and removing the eye shield.

Recently, a gel and a self-adhesive patch have become available (7). The gel was significantly better when compared with EMLA (8).

Lidocaine is used as a 4% spray solution by dentists, otolaryngologists, urologists, and others for either superficial procedures or for laryngoscopy and other endoscopic procedures. Methemoglobinemia has been observed after mucosal application, but appears to be very rare (9).

There is also a *lidocaine patch* (Lidoderm), which is used to alleviate the pain of injection (10). Postzosteric neuralgia was successfully treated with a lidocaine patch (11).

A new liposomal *lidocaine 4% cream* is marketed as ELA-Max and is said to work within about 30 to 45 minutes (12,13).

Lidocaine can be applied via iontophoresis: a sponge soaked with lidocaine is applied to intact skin, and a DC current applied to electrodes over the anes-thetic. The onset of anesthesia is within 10 minutes, and the duration of appli-cation is approximately 15 minutes. The penetration depth is 1 to 2 cm. It is said to be as effective as EMLA cream.

Topical anesthesia became much more efficient with the invention of a *eutectic mixture of lidocaine and prilocaine (EMLA)* (14). This preparation has to be applied generously under occlusion for 1 to 2 hours in adults and 30 to 60 minutes in children, depending on the thickness of the skin, particularly the horny layer. Probably because of the potentiating effect of local anesthetics to endogenous catecholamines, a blanching effect develops that usually indicates that the drug is now working and a superficial anesthesia is achieved. It allows very superficial surgical procedures to be carried out within a time frame of 30 to 45 minutes, but has also been used to reduce postoperative pain in newborns after circumcision (15).

Prilocaine absorption has been observed to cause methemoglobinemia in rare instances in children.

In order to overcome the disadvantage of long-time application and thus delaying surgery or venipuncture for up to two hours, other alternatives were sought. A recent development is a *eutectic mixture of lidocaine and tetracaine,* each 7% in concentration. In a special carrier, it can be applied on the skin and after drying forms a film that can be peeled off (S-Caine, ZARS, Utah, UT, U.S.). No occlusion is necessary. The application time is approximately 30 to 45 minutes (16–21). A self-warming patch is also active within approximately 30 to 45 minutes (22–24).

Topical anesthetics have gained wide acceptance in dermatologic surgery, but also in pediatrics and wherever there is unbalanced fear of a needle prick.

CRYOANESTHESIA

Cold has long been known to produce analgesia. The first agent used was chloroethyl (monochlorethan), which is, however, no longer used because of its potential toxicity when inhaled. In fact, when inhaled in larger quantities, an accidental general anesthesia can occur. Dichlorotetrafluoroethan is not metabolized and almost nontoxic. It allows rapid curettage operations or incisions of furuncles to be performed painlessly. Recently, short sprays of liquid nitrogen were proposed for reducing the pain when injecting botulinum toxin into the palms of the hands for the treatment of palmar hyperhidrosis.

LOCAL ANESTHETICS

The most commonly used agents used for infiltration local anesthesia in dermatologic surgery are listed in Table 3. They are again listed according to their duration of action in Table 4.

Mixtures or combinations of local anesthetics are sometimes used to provide a rapid onset and a prolonged duration of action. However, the possibility of additive toxicity must be considered when such combinations are used.

ESTER-TYPE ANESTHETICS

Procaine

Molecular weight: Procaine hydrochloride 272.78
pK_a: 8.9
Lipid solubility: Low
Protein binding: Very low
Biotransformation: Metabolized to PABA; hydrolyzed primarily in the
    plasma and, to a much lesser extent, in the liver, by cholinesterases
Half-life: 30 to 50 seconds (adults); 54 to 114 seconds (neonates)
Onset of action: Intermediate
Duration of action: Short (30 to 60 minutes).

Relative toxicity 1: Procaine is the standard against which the toxicity
of other local anesthetics is compared
Infiltration anesthesia: Solution of 0.5–2%
Usual dose: 250 to 800 mg; maximal dose: 1 gram
FDA pregnancy category C

Procaine was synthesized in 1904. It soon gained widespread popularity, but it
was also noted that allergies were relatively frequent. Today, it is mainly used
for small interventions because of its short duration of action, for so-called
neural therapy and as a "cure" against aging processes.

Table 3 Most Commonly Used Local Anesthetic Agents in Dermatologic Surgery

Local anesthetic Brand name	Onset	Tolerability Recommended maximum dose without/with adrenaline	Toxicity	Duration of action (min) without/with adrenaline
Lidocaine Xylocaine	3–5 min	Good 300 mg^a/500 mg	Low	Short–medium (30–120/60–400)
Mepivacaine Scandicain	3–5 min	Good 300 mg	Low	Medium (30–120/60–400)
Prilocaine Xylonest	2–3 min	Good 400 mg^a/600 mg	Low	Medium (30–120/60–400)
Ropivacaine Naropin	3–5 min	Very good	Low	Long
Bupivacaine Marcaine, Carbostesine	5 min	Good 175 mg/225 mg	Medium	Very long (120–240/240–480)
Articaine Ultracaine	2–5 min	Good	Medium	Medium
Etidocaine	3–5 min	300 mg		Long (200/240–360)
Procaine Novocaine	>5 min	Medium 500 mg/600 mg (risk of allergy)	Low	Short (15–30/30–90)
Chloroprocaine Nesacaine	Rapid	Good 800 mg/1000 mg	Low	Short (30–60/NA)
Tetracaine Pantocaine	Variable	Low 100 mg/NA	High	Long (120–240/240–480)

^{a}Considerably higher doses are used for tumescence local anesthesia.

Chloroprocaine

Molecular weight: Chloroprocaine hydrochloride 307.22 pK_a: 9
Biotransformation: Metabolized to a PABA derivative
Half-life: 19 to 26 seconds (adults); 41 to 45 seconds (neonates)
Onset of action: Rapid
Duration of action: Variable depending on tissue characteristics (30 to 60 minutes)
FDA pregnancy category C
Chloroprocaine as an ester-type local anesthetic, though having a longer duration of action than procaine, is not widely used in dermatologic surgery.

Table 4 Amide-Type Local Anesthetics Listed According to Their Duration of Action

Short-acting amide anesthetics

Local lidocaine (xylocaine) 1% or 2%
- Onset: 2 min
- Duration: 1.5–2 hr
- Max dose: 4 mg/kg to 280 mg (14 mL 2%, 28 mL 1%) for infiltration, up to 35 mg/kg for tumescence anesthesia

Mepivacaine (Carbocaine, Scandicaine) 1%
- Onset: 3–5 min
- Duration: 1.5–2 hr
- Max dose: 4 mg/kg up to 280 mg (28 mL)

Prilocaine (Citanest) 1%
- Onset: 2 min
- Duration: 1 hr
- Max dose: 7 mg/kg up to 500 mg (50 mL)

Long-acting amide anesthetics

Lidocaine with epinephrine 1:100,000 or 1:200,000
- Onset: 2 min
- Duration: 2–6 hr
- Maximal dose: 7 mg/kg corresponding to 500 mg (25 mL 2%, 50 mL 1%)

Bupivacaine (Marcaine) 0.25%
- Onset: 5 min
- Duration: 2–4 hr
- Maximal dose: 2.5 mg/kg corresponding to 175 mg (50 mL)

Etidocaine (Duranest) 0.5% or 1%
- Maximal dose: 4 mg/kg corresponding to 280 mg (25 mL 1%, 50 mL 0.5%)

Ropivacaine

Tetracaine

Molecular weight: Tetracaine hydrochloride 300.83
pK_a: 8.2
Lipid solubility: High
Protein binding: High
Biotransformation: Metabolized to a PABA derivative by plasma esterases
Onset of action: Rapid
Duration of action: Intermediate to long (1 to >3 hours)
Relative toxicity (compared to procaine): 10
FDA pregnancy category C
Maximal dose when injected locally in adults: 75 mg

A premedication with either a barbiturate or atropine is sometimes advisable. Because of its toxicity, tetracaine is only rarely used for infiltration or nerve block anesthesia in dermatology.

AMIDE-TYPE ANESTHETICS

In general, amide-type local anesthetics have many advantages over ester-type ones. Particularly their sensitization potential is much less, and true allergies to amide-type anesthetics are very rare.

Lidocaine (also Lignocaine)

2-(Diethylamino)-N-(2,6-dimethylphenyl) acetamide
Molecular weight: Lidocaine hydrochloride 288.82
pK_a: 7.9
Lipid solubility: Medium
Protein binding: Moderate to high (60–90%), primarily to α_1-acid glycoprotein
Biotransformation: Metabolic breakdown in the liver to xylidides, which are toxic but less so than the parent compound. One metabolite— monoethylglycine xylide—is active. There is some concern that large amounts of xylidides might have a carcinogenic potential. The metabolites are excreted renally; less than 10% unchanged, 3–4% as the active metabolite. Hypotension may decrease the liver metabolism because of decreased blood supply to the liver and slow down lidocaine clearance.
Half-life: 1.5 to 2 hours (adults); 3.2 hours (neonates)
Onset of action: Rapid
Duration of action: Intermediate (1 to 3 hours)
Relative toxicity (compared to procaine): 2
FDA pregnancy category B
Usual dose in adults: 200 mg/day; however, in tumescent anesthesia, doses of up to 35 to 50 mg/kg body weight were shown to be safe with peak

serum concentrations not exceeding the allowed concentrations. There is a considerable interindividual variation in plasma concentrations after injection of the same dose because of variable α_1-glycoprotein levels. Signs of toxicity may appear with 5 to 5.5 µg of lidocaine/mL plasma. Lidocaine penetrates into the cerebrospinal fluid and crosses the placental barrier with fetal blood concentration reaching roughly half that of the mother. Commonly, the lidocaine solution for infiltration is 1–2%; however, up to 5% can be used safely if necessary.

Lidocaine is certainly the most commonly used local anesthetic in dermatologic surgery and has an excellent safety report. It can be effectively used for all sorts of local anesthesia. It is also used in cardiology as antiarrhythmic drug as an intravenous infusion. In dermatology, a case of intravenous lidocaine treatment for chronic cholangitic pruritus in an AIDS patient was described.

However, there are some possible drug interactions that may cause problems during or after the local infiltration. Cimetidine and β-blockers may impair the metabolism of lidocaine, whereas enzyme inductors such as barbiturates, carbamazepine, phenytoin, or rifampicin may accelerate it. The cardiodepressive action of antiarrhythmic drugs may be increased.

The most severe side effects reported are sudden death that may have been due to the added conservatives or vasoconstrictors, cardiac arrest, bronchospasm, and anaphylactic shock (after intravenous injection).

Contraindications are myasthenia, supraventricular arrhythmia, and porphyrias.

Mepivacaine

1,2′,6′,-Trimethyl piperidine-2-carboxy anilide hydrochloride
Molecular weight: Mepivacaine hydrochloride 282.81
pK_a: 7.6
Lipid solubility: Medium
Protein binding: High
Half-life: 1.9 to 3.2 hours (adults); 9 hours (neonates)
Onset of action: Rapid to intermediate
Duration of action: Intermediate (1 to 3 hours)
Relative toxicity (compared to procaine): 2
FDA pregnancy category C
Usual dose for local injection: 50 to 200 mg

Mepivacaine is as safe as lidocaine. It can be used for almost all cases in dermatologic surgery that are suitable for local anesthesia.

Although there is some evidence that systemic toxicity may be more likely to occur in pediatric patients, appropriate studies performed to date with mepivacaine have not demonstrated pediatrics-specific problems that would limit the use of the medication in children.

Mepivavaine has recently also been used for tumescent anesthesia (see below).

A patient who tolerated lidocaine well developed a pigmented, fixed drug eruption on four occasions after mepivacaine.

Prilocaine

Molecular weight: Prilocaine hydrochloride 256.78
pK_a: 7.9
Lipid solubility: Medium
Protein binding: Moderate
Biotransformation: Metabolized mainly in the liver, but also by kidney
   and lung tissue
Half-life: 1.6 hours
Onset of action: Rapid
Duration of action: Intermediate (1–3 hours)
Relative toxicity (compared to procaine): 1.7
FDA pregnancy category B

The resorption after injection depends on the vascularization of the tissue and is therefore dependent on the site, tissue conditions, blood pressure, etc. The metabolism is hepatic and to some degree renal with formation of metabolites, particularly ortho-toluidin, which cause methemoglobinemia in higher doses. The metabolites are, at least in part, excreted by the kidney.

Except for its potential to cause methemoglobinemia that does not reach considerable levels after common doses, prilocaine is very safe with the lowest relative toxicity after procaine. It can be used for infiltration anesthesia and nerve blocks as well as tumescent anesthesia. Methemoglobinemia may cause concern when large amounts of prilocaine are given in tumescent anesthesia (see below).

Etidocaine (Duranest ^{R})

($\pm$)-(N-Ethyl-propylamino)-2-dimethyl-2′,6′butyranilide;
   ($\pm$)-[(N-ethyl-propylamino)-2 butyroxy]-2,6-xylidide
Molecular weight: 276.42
pK_a: 7.74
Lipid solubility: High
Protein binding: Very high
Half-life: 2.5 hours (adults); 4 to 8 hours (neonates)
Onset of action: Rapid
Duration of action: Long (3 to 10 hours). The addition of epinephrine does
   not prolong the duration of analgesia but allows maintenance of lower
   plasma concentrations of the anesthetic. It also significantly shortens
   the onset time of a sensory blockade.
FDA pregnancy category B
Elimination: Less than 10% of a dose may be excreted unchanged

Etidocaine (Duranest) is available as a plain 1% (pH, 4–5) and 1% and 1.5% with adrenaline 1:200,000 solution (pH, 3–4.5), the latter 2 containing 0.5 mg sodium metabisulfite and 0.2 mg citric acid/mL.

Potential drug interactions with etidocaine are not substantially different from other amide-type anesthetics:

- Blood thinners such as warfarin
- Antidepressive drugs: Monoamine oxidase inhibitors (MAOIs) such as isocarboxacid and phenelzine
- Guanadrel
- Guanethidine
- Medicines for high blood pressure
- Drugs that improve muscle strength or tone, for conditions like myasthenia gravis
- Mecamylamine

Etidocaine is a long-acting local anesthetic that is well tolerated not only for nerve blocks but also for infiltration anesthesia.

Articaine (Carticaine)

Articaine is an amide-type local anesthetic with an ester linkage and a thiophene ring.

4-Methyl-3-(2-propylaminopropionamido)-2-carboxyl-thiophene hydrochloride
Molecular weight: Articaine 284.38
Half-life:1.2 hours
Onset of action: Rapid (within 1 to 6 minutes)
Duration of action: Intermediate (1 to 3 hours)
Articaine is inactivated by ester hydrolysis via plasma carboxyesterase
  to articainic acid. Approximately 5–10% of articaine is metabolized
  by liver microsome P450 isoenzymes to articainic acid.
FDA pregnancy category C

Articaine was originally developed for use in dentistry. However, it was found that its unique chemical structure—though being an amide-type anesthetic—allows the body to rapidly inactivate articaine that is taken up by the circulation. Since this is a fast process, the drug may be reinjected within a relatively short period, if necessary. It is now used for nerve blocks and infiltrations also outside dental surgery. Recently, it was used for tumescent anesthesia and all studies showed that it is as effective for liposuction, varicose veins, and skin tumor surgery as the classical lidocaine or prilocaine solutions (25–28) (see below).

Bupivaine

1-Butyl-2′,6′-dimethyl-piperidine-2-carboxanilide hydrochloride
Molecular weight: Bupivacaine hydrochloride 342.91
Lipid solubility: High

Protein binding: Very high (95%), mainly acidic α_1-glycoprotein and albumin
Half-life: 3.5 hours (1.5 to 5.5) in adults; 8.1 to 14 hours in neonates
Onset of action: Intermediate
FDA pregnancy category C
Main indications: Infiltration anesthesia, nerve block
Elimination: Renal
Bupivacaine resorption from the injection site into the blood is slow.
After peridural or pericaudal injection of 125 to 150 mg of bupivacain
    hydrochloride, peak plasma levels of 0.45 to 1.25 µg/mL are reached in
    30 to 45 minutes.
Tissue distribution: Lipid-rich tissues such as brain, heart, and lung, but
    also subcutaneous adipose tissue, retain considerable amounts of
    bupivacaine. It can pass into the cerebrospinal liquor. Because of its
    high protein binding, there is almost no risk of crossing the placental
    barrier and little distribution into breast milk.
It is metabolized by a cytochrome 450–dependent mono-oxygenase in
    the liver to pipecolyl xylidine and pipecoline acid.
The metabolites are mainly eliminated by the kidney, 5–6% in the unchanged
    form.
Interaction with cimetidine.
Prolonged cardiovascular depression and arrhythmias have been reported.
    The cardiotoxicity of bupivacaine may be increased if the patient
    experiences hypothermia, hyponatremia, hyperkalemia, or myocardial
    ischemia. Concomitant use of halothane may cause increased cardio-
    toxicity of bupivacaine.
One case of allergic rhinoconjunctivitis 30 minutes after subcutaneous injection
    of a test dose was described in a patient who reported an allergy.
Acute intermittent porphyria is a contraindication.

Levobupivacaine (Chirocaine)

(S)-1-Butyl-2-piperidylformo-2′, 6′-xylidide
Molecular weight: 324.9
pK_a:8.1
Lipid solubility: High
Protein binding: Very high
Half-life: 1.3 hours
Onset of action: Immediate to slow
Duration of action: Medium to long
Elimination: Completely in metabolized form
Metabolism: In the liver by cytochrome P450 (CYP) 3A4 and CYP1A2
    isoforms to desbutyl levobupivacaine and 3-hydroxy levobupivacaine,
    respectively
Drug interactions and/or related problems: Interactions may occur with
    CYP3A4 inducers (such as phenytoin, phenobarbital, rifampin),
    CYP3A4 inhibitors (azole antifungals, protease inhibitors, macrolide

antibiotics), CYP1A2 inducers (omeprazole), and CYP1A2 inhibitors (clarithromycin)

FDA pregnancy category B

Usual adult dose: Moderate to complete peripheral nerve block; 75 to 150 mg or 1 to 2 mg/kg (30 mL/kg or 0.4 mL/kg) as a 0.25% and 0.5% solution

Local infiltration: 150 mg (60 mL) as a 0.25% solution

Strength(s) usually available: Without preservative, 0.25% (2.5 mg/mL) [*Chirocaine* (preservative free)], 0.5% (5 mg/mL) [*Chirocaine* (preservative free)], 0.75% (7.5 mg/mL) [*Chirocaine* (preservative free)]

Levobupivacaine is the S-enantiomer of bupivacaine and less cardiotoxic than its parent compound.

Levobupivacaine and ropivacaine are equally effective in patients undergoing an axillary brachial plexus block.

Ropivacaine

S(–)-1-Propyl-2′-6′-pipecoloxylidide hydrochloride

Protein binding: Very high (95%)

Half-life: 1.8 hours

Elimination: 86% renal

Toxicity: The S-enantiomer is much less cardiotoxic than bupivacaine (between lidocaine and bupivacaine); its effect is only slightly less

Usual dose in adults: Up to 200 mg as a 0.75% solution for surgical anesthesias (same dose, but as a 0.2% solution for the treatment of acute pain conditions)

Metabolism: Completely metabolized by the liver by aromatic hydroxylation yielding 3-hydroxy-ropivacaine and 2-hydroxy-methyl-ropivacaine

Ropivaine is mainly used for regional anesthesia, but can also be used for infiltration anesthesia. It comes as a 0.2%, 0.75%, or 1% injection solution. The low concentration is for large area anesthesia (29–31).

Ropivacaine appears to have a mild intrinsic vasoconstrictor activity (32).

We have excellent experience with ropivacaine 1% for transthecal blocks in nail surgery. It lasts many hours, sometimes more than 24 hours, ensuring complete absence of pain.

A summary of pharmacologic and pharmacokinetic properties of important local aneshetics is given in Table 5.

ADDITIONS TO LOCAL ANESTHETICS

Solutions of local anesthetics often contain additives. The most common ones are preservatives, among which parabens are the most commonly added. They are, like the ester-type local anesthetics, derivatives of PABA and may cross-react with the anesthetics.

Table 5 Pharmacology/Pharmacokinetics of Local Anesthetics

Drug	pK_a	Lipid solubility (pH 7.4)	Protein binding	Half-life adult/ neonate	Onset of action[a]	Duration of action[b]	Relative toxicity[c]
Articaine	7.8	High	Medium (60–80%)	1.2 hr	Rapid (1–6 min)	Intermediate (1 hr)	
Bupivacaine	8.1	High	Very high	3.5 hr/8.1–14 hr	Intermediate to slow	Long[d]	
Chloroprocaine	9			19–26 sec/ 41–45 sec	Rapid	Short	
Etidocaine	7.74	High	Very high	2.5 hr/4–8 hr	Rapid	Long	
Levobupivacaine	8.1	High	Very high	1.3 hr	Immediate to slow	Short to long	
Lidocaine	7.9	Medium	Moderate to high	1.5–2 hr/3.2 hr	Rapid[e]	Intermediate	2
Mepivacaine	7.6	Medium	High	1.9–3.2 hr/9 hr	Rapid to intermediate	Intermediate	2
Prilocaine	7.9	Medium	Moderate	1.6 hr	Rapid	Intermediate	1.7
Procaine	8.9	Low	Very low	30–50 sec/ 54–114 sec	Intermediate	Short	1
Tetracaine	8.2	High	High		Rapid	Intermediate to long	10

[a]Influenced by the site, route, and technique of administration; dosage (volume and concentration) administered; pH at injection site; physical characteristics, such as lipid solubility, molecular size, and pK_a of the individual anesthetic; and individual patient.

[b]Short = 30–60 min; Intermediate = 1–3 hr; Long = 3–10 hr. Influenced by factors affecting rate of clearance from the injection site and individual patient.

[c]As compared with procaine (the least toxic of these agents).

[d]Via nerve block, may produce analgesia for considerably longer than 10 hr.

[e]Adjustment of pH with 1 mEq (1 mmol) of sodium bicarbonate per 10 mL may increase the onset of conduction blocks (lidocaine hydrochloride injection, lidocaine and epinephrine injection, or mepivacaine hydrochloride injection).

Other additives are vasoconstrictors, buffers, spreading agents, and more rarely steroids as anti-inflammatory agents. Opioids and other analgesics were sometimes added to prolong the action of the local anesthesia in knee and other surgeries, but they are not used in dermatologic surgery.

Vasoconstrictors

Vasoconstrictors are added to local anesthetic injections to decrease the rate of local clearance of the local anesthetic. Local anesthetic injections containing a vasoconstrictor generally have the same indications as the corresponding local anesthetic injection without a vasoconstrictor. However, additional precautions pertinent to the use of a vasoconstrictor must be considered.

Vasoconstrictors are often advantageous because, except for cocaine, the local anesthesia causes vasodilation by a direct effect on the neuromuscular stimulation, thus producing vasodilation. They also decrease the absorption of the local anesthetic into the circulation, thus prolonging its action.

Vasoconstrictors decrease the rate of local clearance of the local anesthetic, thereby reducing the risk of systemic toxic reactions, prolonging the anesthetic effect, increasing the frequency of complete conduction blocks at low anesthetic concentrations, and permitting larger maximum single doses of anesthetic to be administered. Epinephrine 1:200,000 is the most commonly used vasoconstrictor for most purposes; levonordefrin, norepinephrine, and phenylephrine may also be used.

Adrenaline and Other Substances with α-Adrenergic Activity

Adrenaline (epinephrine) is usually added in a concentration of 1:100,000 or 1:200,000, depending on the location and the need to decrease bleeding. For tumescent anesthesia, 1 mg is added to 1 L of tumescent fluid. High concentrations or larger amounts may cause cardiovascular and CNS side effects. These are uncommon when noradrenaline (norepinephrine) is used (33), but it is slightly less potent than adrenaline. These catecholamine vasoconstrictors are physiologic substances and are followed by a physiologic post-ischemic hyperemia. This may cause delayed postoperative bleeding. Exact hemostasis is therefore necessary when using these substances.

Adrenaline (epinephrine) and levonordefrin have α- and a weaker β-adrenergic activity, which is very weak for noradrenaline (norepinephrine). Because of their β-adrenergic activity, they may cause cardiac stimulation, resulting in increased heart rate, contractility, conduction velocity, and irritability. Also, when used for obstetrical anesthesia, vasoconstrictors with β-adrenergic activity may decrease the intensity of uterine contractions and prolong labor.

Phenylephrine is also used as a (weak) vasoconstrictor in conjunction with local anesthesia; it has only α-adrenergic activity and does not have these additional effects. Ornipressin is a strong vasocontrictor and devoid of cardiac side effects, but its long duration may interfere with wound healing.

SODIUM BICARBONATE

The infiltration of acidic solutions is more painful and addition of sodium bicarbonate as a buffer was repeatedly shown to decrease this pain (34–36). Most local anesthetics have an acidic pH, e.g., lidocaine without adrenaline about 5 to 7, with adrenaline between 3.3 to 5.5. The injection of an acidic local anesthetic into tissue, particularly when it is inflamed or has been recently operated on, is painful. The anesthetics are primarily weakly basic compounds that are lipophilic and have to be transformed into hydrophilic salts to be soluble. The solutions commonly have a pH of 4 to 5 (6). These solutions are more stable, but tissue irritating (37). Solutions containing adrenaline are usually even more acidic to prolong their stability. However, to achieve an effective analgesia, the anesthetic should be injected with a physiologic pH and sufficient buffer capacity, allowing the then undissociated molecules to cross the lipophilic membrane of the nerve fibers. Inflamed tissue has a pH of approximately 6, thus slowing down the penetration of the anesthetic into the nerve. Addition of 1 mEq of sodium bicarbonate 8.4% to 100 mL of anesthetic solution (10 mL NaHCO$_3$ 8.4% per 1 L) reduces injection pain considerably. Sodium bicarbonate is freshly added just before injection because adrenaline will slowly decompose in an alkaline pH. For every 10 mL of lidocaine with adrenaline, 1 mL of 8.4% sodium bicarbonate is added. Adrenaline in the neutralized local anesthetic agent degrades at a rate of about 25% per week.

Adrenaline can also be used for digital anesthesia and in other acral regions provided there is no obvious peripheral circulatory disease (38–40).

Another advantage of the addition of bicarbonate is that it increases the intrinsic antibacterial action of lidocaine and some other local anesthetics (41).

Benzyl Alcohol

Benzyl alcohol is used as a bacteriostatic agent in many injection solutions. It has an intrinsic local anesthetic action, which, however, is relatively weak and lasts for only about 2 to 5 minutes. Both lidocaine and adrenaline can prolong its effects (42). The injection of saline containing 0.9% benzyl alcohol is essentially painless. Because the pH of this bacteriostatic saline is slightly acidic, it was speculated that the pH is not the only factor responsible for pain of injection.

Hyaluronidase

Good spreading properties of a local anesthetic solution mean that it diffuses better in scar tissue and reaches a wider area and that specific nerve blocks need less accuracy. Hyaluronidase splits up hyaluronic acid into smaller molecule parts. This facilitates rapid diffusion of the anesthetic, thus minimizing anatomic distortion of the infiltrated area (43). Commonly, 50 units are added to 10 mL of anesthetic fluid. Its main indications are local anesthesias around the eye or peripheral nerve blocks.

SOLUTIONS FOR TUMESCENT LOCAL ANESTHESIA
AND SUBCUTANEOUS INFUSION ANESTHESIA

Tumescent anesthesia was developed for liposuction by the dermatologist J. A. Klein and published for the first time in 1987 (44). His invention was initiated by the increasing need of U.S. dermatologic surgeons to perform their activities in outpatient settings and under local anesthesia. It had been shown that large volumes of fluids facilitate liposuction (45). Klein's ingenious thought was to combine Illouz's wet technique with the common local infiltration anesthesia. He further studied his tumescent anesthesia solution and its toxicity and, by careful and meticulous studies, found out that the total and relative dose of lidocaine could be increased sevenfold (46). It was later shown that the dose could even be increased to 50 to 55 mg/kg body weight (47), though in relatively thin patients, 45 mg/kg is better not exceeded (48). Investigations in the United States proved that tumescent anesthesia is extremely safe in dermatologic outpatient liposuction surgery (49), far safer than under general anesthesia. The advantages of tumescent anesthesia did not take long to get recognized for noncosmetic dermatologic surgery. It is now standard in most dermatologic surgery divisions to perform large excision, wound repairs, vein surgery, etc., under tumescent anesthesia (50–52). The large volume tightens the tissue and facilitates the harvesting of split thickness grafts or hair-bearing grafts for hair transplantation (53). In fact, there is virtually no dermatologic surgical procedure that cannot be performed under tumescent local anesthesia. New mixtures, lower concentrations, and more gentle application modes of tumescent solutions were and are still being developed (54) (Table 6).

Table 6 Klein's Tumescent Anesthesia Formulations: Only the Lidocaine Amounts Are Decreasing, Whereas Adrenaline and Sodium Bicarbonate Depend on the Volume of the Solution

Substance	Amount for 1 L		Amount for 100 mL	
Lidocaine 0.1%				
Lidocaine 1%	100 mL	1000 mg	10 mL	100 mg
Adrenaline	1 mL	1 mg	0.1 mL	0.1 mg
$NaHCO_3$	12.5 mL	12.5 mEq	1.25 mL	1.25 mEq
NaCl 0.9%	1000 mL	1000 mL	100 mL	100 mL
Lidocaine 0.05%				
Lidocaine 1%	50 mL	500 mg	5 mL	50 mg
Adrenaline	1 mL	1 mg	0.1 mL	0.1 mg
$NaHCO_3$	12.5 mL	12.5 mEq	1.25 mL	1.25 mEq
NaCl 0.9%	1000 mL	1000 mL	100 mL	100 mL
Lidocaine 0.01%				
Lidocaine 1%	10 mL	100 mg	1 mL	10 mg
Adrenaline	1 mL	1 mg	0.1 mL	0.1 mg
$NaHCO_3$	12.5 mL	12.5 mEq	1.25 mL	1.25 mEq
NaCl 0.9%	1000 mL	1000 mL	100 mL	100 mL

Table 7 Preparation of Solutions for Subcutaneous Infusion Anesthesia

Concentration (%)	Amount	Vasoconstrictor
0.3	400 mL Ringer's solution 50 mL prilocaine 2% 50 mL ropivacaine 1%	Adrenaline 0.5 mg
0.15	425 mL Ringer's solution 50 mL prilocaine 1% 25 mL ropivacaine 1%	Adrenaline 0.5 mg
0.08	460 mL Ringer's solution 25 mL prilocaine 1% 15 mL ropivacaine 1%	Adrenaline 0.5 mg

Source: From Refs. 56,57.

Since about 10 years, prilocaine has been used mainly in Germany because of its considerably lower toxicity compared with lidocaine, except for methemoglobin formation after large amounts (54). Mepivacaine has also been used successfully (55). Recently, articaine was introduced into tumescent anesthesia because of its property of being rapidly metabolized in the blood circulation into articainic acid, which is no longer toxic (25,27,28).

Slow infusion anesthesia is a variant of tumescent local anesthesia. Using 30-gauge needles and injection pumps, an almost painless subcutaneous infusion of a mixture of prilocaine and ropivacaine is used (56,57) (Table 7). This technique, which allows very slow infusion rates that avoid the pain from pressure of rapid injection, is also particularly useful for young children and provides a painless area for more than five hours (58). We have found ropivacaine to be very useful for varicose vein surgery and large excisions with flap repairs (59).

CONCLUSION

There are many local anesthetics for use in dermatologic surgery that are safe, efficacious, and convenient both for the dermatologist and the patient.

REFERENCES

1. Malamed SF, Sykes P, Kubota Y, et al. Local anesthesia: a review. Anesth Pain Control Dent 1992; 1:11–24.
2. Malamed S F. Local anesthetics: dentistry's most important drugs. JADA 1994; 125:1571–1576.
3. Borehard U. Zahnärztliche Therapie während der Schwangerschaft. Proceedings, European Meeting on Sedation and Anaesthesia in Dentistry, 1992, 2–4.

4. Willershausen-Zönnchen B. Zahnärztliche Behandlung in der Schwangerschaft. Dtsch Zahnärztl Z 1994; 49:653.

5. Wildsmith JAW, Strichartz GR. Local anaesthetic drugs—a historical perspective. Br J Anaesth 1984; 56:937–939.

6. Fink BR. Leaves and needles: the introduction of surgical local anesthesia. Anesthesiology 1985; 63:77–83.

7. McCafferty DF, Woolfson AD, Handley J, et al. Effect of percutaneous local anaesthetics on pain reduction during pulse dye laser treatment of portwine stains. Br J Anaesth 1997; 78:286–289.

8. McCafferty DF, Woolfson AD, Moss GP. Novel bioadhesive delivery system for percutaneous local anaesthesia. Br J Anaesth 2000; 84:456–458.

9. O'Donohue WJ Jr., Moss LM, Angelillo VA. Acute methemoglobinemia induced by topical benzocaine and lidocaine. Arch Intern Med 1980; 140:1508–1509.

10. Onguchi T, Takano Y, Dogru M, et al. Lidocaine tape (Penles) reduces the pain of botulinum toxin injection for Meige syndrome. Am J Ophthalmol 2004; 138:654–655.

11. Comer AM, Lamb HM. Lidocaine patch. Drugs 2000; 59:245–249.

12. Goldman RD. ELA-Max: a new topical lidocaine formulation. Ann Pharmacother 2004; 38:892–894.

13. Shin SC, Cho CW, Yang KH. Development of lidocaine gels for enhanced local anesthetic action. Int J Pharm 2004; 287(1-2):73–78.

14. Juhlin L, Evers H. EMLA: a new topical anesthetic. Adv Dermatol 1990; 5:75–92.

15. Taddio A, Stevens B, Craig K, et al. Efficacy and safety of lidocaine-prilocaine cream forpain during circumcision. N Engl J Med 1997; 336:1197–1201.

16. Bryan HA, Alster TS. The S-Caine peel: a novel topical anesthetic for cutaneous laser surgery. Dermatol Surg. 2002; 28:999–1003; discussion 1003.

17. Alster TS, Lupton JR. Evaluation of a novel topical anesthetic agent for cutaneous laser resurfacing: a randomized comparison study. Dermatol Surg 2002; 28: 1004–1006; discussion 1006.

18. Doshi SN, Friedman PM, Marquez DK, et al. Thirty-minute application of the S-Caine peel prior to nonablative laser treatment. Dermatol Surg 2003; 29:1008–1011.

19. Chen JZ, Alexiades-Armenakas MR, Bernstein LJ, et al. Two randomized, double-blind, placebo-controlled studies evaluating the S-Caine Peel for induction of local anesthesia before long-pulsed Nd:YAG laser therapy for leg veins. Dermatol Surg 2003; 29:1012–1018.

20. Jih MH, Friedman PM, Sadick N, et al. 60-minute application of S-Caine Peel prior to 1,064 nm long-pulsed Nd:YAG laser treatment of leg veins. Lasers Surg Med 2004; 34:446–450.

21. Sethna NF, Verghese ST, Hannallah RS, et al. A randomized controlled trial to evaluate S-Caine patch for reducing pain associated with vascular access in children. Anesthesiology 2005; 102:403–408.

22. Berman B, Flores J, Pariser D, et al. Self-warming lidocaine/tetracaine patch effectively and safely induces local anesthesia during minor dermatologic procedures. Dermatol Surg 2005; 31:135–138.

23. Shomaker TS, Zhang J, Love G, et al. Evaluating skin anesthesia after administration of a local anesthetic system consisting of an S-Caine patch and a controlled heat-aided drug delivery (CHADD) patch in volunteers. Clin J Pain 2000; 16: 200–204.

24. Long CP, McCafferty DF, Sittlington NM, et al. Randomized trial of novel tetracaine patch to provide local anaesthesia in neonates undergoing venepuncture. Br J Anaesth 2003; 91:514–518.
25. Grossmann M, Sattler G, Pistner H, et al. Pharmacokinetics of articaine hydrochloride in tumescent local anesthesia for liposuction. J Clin Pharmacol 2004; 44:1282–1289.
26. Malamed SF, Gagnon S, Leblanc D. A comparison between articaine HCl and lidocaine HCl in pediatric dental patients. Pediatr Dent 2000; 22:307–311.
27. Bruning G, Rasmussen H, Wolf C, et al. Articain versus Prilocain: Die Lösung der Toxizitätsfrage der Tumeszenzlokalanästhesie? Akt Dermatol 2004; 30:436–437 (abstr.).
28. Fatemi A. Tumeszenzlokalanästhesie mit Articain—die ideale Lösung? Akt Dermatol 2004; 30:437 (abstr).
29. de Jong RH. 1995 Gaston Labat Lecture. Ropivacaine. White knight or dark horse? Reg-Anesth 1995; 20:474–481.
30. Lee A, Fagan D, Lamont M, et al. Disposition kinetics of ropivacaine in humans. Anesth Analg 1989; 69:736–738.
31. Datta S, Camann W, Bader A, et al. Clinical effects and maternal and fetal plasma concentrations of epidural ropivacaine versus bupivacaine for cesarean section. Anesthesiology 1995; 82:1346–1352.
32. Millay DJ, Larrabee WF Jr., Carpenter RL. Vasoconstrictors in facial plastic surgery. Arch Otolaryngol Head Neck Surg 1991; 117:160–163.
33. Haneke E. Noradrenalin statt Adrenalin beim Schock. Dtsch med Wschr 1976; 101:1170.
34. Davis J. Vasoconstrictor for facelifting. Aesthetic Plast Surg 1988; 12:33–34.
35. McKay W, Morris R, Mushlin P. Sodium bicarbonate attenuates pain on skin infiltration with lidocaine, with or without epinephrine. Anesth Analg 1987; 66:572–574.
36. Stewart JH, Cole GW, Klein JA. Neutralized lidocaine with epinephrine for local anesthesia. J Dermatol Surg Oncol 1989; 15:1081–1083.
37. Cheney PR, Molzen G, Tandberg D. The effect of pH buffering on reducing the pain associated with subcutaneous infiltration bupivacaine. Am J Emerg Med 1991; 9:147–148.
38. Krunic AL, Wang LC, Soltani K, et al. Digital anesthesia with epinephrine: an old myth revisited. J Am Acad Dermatol 2004; 51:755–759.
39. Häfner H-M, Röcken M, Breuninger H. Epinephrine-supplemented local anesthetics for ear and nose surgery: clinical use without complications in more than 10,000 surgical procedures. J Dtsch Dermatol Ges 2005; 3:195–199.
40. Haneke E. Lokalanästhesie mit Adrenalinzusatz an Ohr und Nase. Editorial. J Dtsch Dermatol Ges 2005; 3:161–162.
41. Thompson KD, Welykij S, Massa MC. Antibacterial activity of lidocaine in combination with a bicarbonate buffer. J Dermatol Surg Oncol 1993; 19:216–220.
42. Lugo-Janer G, Padial M, Sánchez JL. Less painful alternative for local anesthesia. J Dermatol Surg Oncol 1993; 18:130–135.
43. Lewis-Smith PA. Adjunctive use of hyaluronidase in local anaesthesia. Br J Plast Surg 1986; 39:554–558.
44. Klein JA. The tumescent technique for liposuction surgery. Am J Cosm Surg 1987; 4:263–267.

45. Illouz Y. Body contouring by lipolysis: a 5 year experience with over 3000 cases. Plast Reconstr Surg 1983; 72:511–518.
46. Klein JA. Tumescent technique for regional anesthesia permits lidocaine doses of 35 mg/kg for liposuction. J Dermatol Surg Oncol 1990; 16:248–263.
47. Ostad A, Kageyama N, Moy RL. Tumescent anesthesia with a lidocaine dose of 55 mg/kg is safe in large volume liposuction. Plast Reconstr Surg 1993; 92:1085–1098.
48. Klein JA. Anesthetic formulation of tumescent solutions. Dermatol Clin 1999; 17:751–759.
49. Hanke CW, Bernstein G, Bullock BS. Safety of tumescent liposuctions in 15336 patients—national survey results. Dermatol Surg 1995; 21:459–462.
50. Colemean WP, Klein JA. Use of the tumescent technique for scalp surgery, dermabrasion, and soft tissue reconstruction. J Dermatol Surg Oncol 1992; 18:130–135.
51. Acosta AE. Clinical parameters of tumescent anesthesia in skin cancer reconstructive surgery. Arch Dermatol 1997; 133:451–454.
52. Sattler G. Lokalanästhesie, Regionalanästhesie, Tumeszenzanästhesie: Techniken und Indikationen. Z Hautkr 1998; 73:116.
53. Field LM, Hrabovszky T. Harvesting split-thickness grafts with tumescent anesthesia. Dermatol Surg 1997; 23:62.
54. Sommer B, Sattler G, Hanke CW, (eds.). Tumeszenz-Lokalanästhesie. Berlin: Springer, 1999.
55. Kasten R, Dorfner B. Vergleich der Schmerzhaftigkeit einer Infiltrationsanästhesie mit gepufferten und ungepufferten Lösungen von Mepivacain 1% bei zweizeitigen dermatochirurgischen Eingriffen im Gesicht. In: Augustin M, Peschen M, Petres J. Innovation und Qualität in der operativen Dermatologie. Fortschritte der operativen und onkologischen Dermatologie. Vol 18. Berlin: Congress Compact Verlag, 2003. 45–48.
56. Breuninger H, Wehner-Caroli J. Slow infusion tumescent anesthesia. Dermatol Surg 1998; 24:759–763.
57. Breuninger H, Schimek F, Heeg P. Subcutaneous infusion anesthesia with diluted mixtures of prilocaine and ropivacaine. Langenbecks Arch Surg 2000; 385:284–289.
58. Moehrle M, Breuninger H. Dermatosurgery using subcutaneous infusion anesthesia with prilocaine and ropicavacaine in children. Pediatr Dermatol 2001; 18:469–472.
59. Haneke E. Tumescence anaesthesia for surgery of varicose veins. Przegl Flebol 2006; 14:27–32.

2

Vasoconstrictors: Chemistry, Mode of Action, and Dosage

Paul O. Larson

*Retired, Mohs Surgery Clinic,
University of Wisconsin, Madison,
Wisconsin, U.S.A.*

INTRODUCTION

Vasoconstrictors play a very important role in providing optimal local anesthesia in dermatologic surgery. They first slow the circulation and mobilization of the injected local anesthetic, thus prolonging the effect of the anesthetic. Second, by slowing mobilization of the anesthetic, they reduce the peak blood levels of the anesthetic, which in turn reduces the potential for toxicity from the anesthetic. This also permits administration of larger volumes of anesthetic and more complete anesthetic. Finally, vasoconstrictors provide hemostasis during surgery, which results in a better, faster, and safer surgery.

PHYSIOLOGY OF VASOCONSTRICTION

An understanding of vasoconstrictors requires a brief review of the physiology of vasoconstriction. Contraction of smooth muscles in arterioles and venules is primarily controlled by the autonomic nervous system (automatic controls)—the somatic nerves are controlled by conscious thought (conscious controls). Vasoconstriction is largely controlled by the autonomic system and to a lesser extent by vasoactive peptides. Direct reflexes affect vasoconstriction to a very limited extent.

Autonomic Nervous System

The autonomic system is divided into two major subdivision based primarily on where the systems are located—the *parasympathetic* is organized around the craniosacral regions, and the *sympathetic* system organized around the thoracolumbar regions (1).

The parasympathetic system is most frequently associated with release of the neurotransmitter acetylcholine, which are then called *cholinergic* receptors (1).

The sympathetic system, which is associated with the "fight or flight" reactions, largely comprises postganglionic fibers, which release the neurotransmitter norepinephrine, and are called *adrenergic* (1). The sympathetic system is largely responsible for control of vascular tone, vasoconstriction, and vasodilatation.

The sympathetic nervous system responds to a variety of stimuli mediated by the central nervous system to control normal homeostasis. The CNS activates the sympathetic system following cold stress, exercise, postural hypotension, or fear (fight or flight) (2).

Adrenal System

The adrenal gland also helps mediate vascular homeostasis by releasing adrenergic compounds from the adrenal gland into the blood stream, e.g., epinephrine (80–90%) and norepinephrine (10–20%) (3). These adrenergic compounds are activated by anxiety, stress, hypoxia, or hypoglycemia.

Neurotransmitters

Norepinephrine is the primary neurotransmitter of the sympathetic nervous system. It is released primarily from the sympathetic nerve fibers; however, about 20% is secreted from the adrenal gland and is quickly bound to albumin. Blood levels are normally from 100–350 ng/mL (4).

Epinephrine has similar actions to norepinephrine, but all of it is secreted from the adrenal medulla. It is quickly bound to albumin. The normal blood level is 20–50 ng/mL (4).

Cotransmitters also regulate the autonomic system. Dopamine is an important co-transmitter, which regulates renal blood flow. Other co-transmitters include ATP, nitric oxide, serotonin, substance P, and vasoactive intestinal peptide (VIP) (1). Neuropeptide Y causes long-lasting vasoconstriction (1). The roll of co-transmitters is not as well understood as the adrenergic transmitters.

Adrenergic Receptors

Adrenergic receptors are divided into two major categories—the α and β receptors, which again are subdivided. Some organs have only one of the

Table 1 Adrenergic Receptors and the Results of Their Activation

Receptor	Results
α1	Vasoconstriction
	Increases renin release, sphincter tone, uterine contractions, glycogenolysis, and gluconeogenesis
	Decreases GI motility
α2	Vasoconstriction
	Modulates large vessel tone by opposing α1 receptor vasoconstriction and norepinephrine release
	Increases sphincter tone and uterine contractions
	Decreases GI motility, insulin, and glucagon levels
β1	Increases myocardial contractility and heart rate
	Increases renin release, glycogenolysis, gluconeogenesis and lipolysis
β2	Vasodilation of skeletal and vascular smooth muscle
	Bronchiodilation
	Increases renin release, insulin levels and glucagon levels, and increases glycogenolysis and gluconeogenesis

Source: From Refs. 81, 82.

receptors and others have both. These receptors can be selectively stimulated or blocked by the various neurotransmitting agents (Table 1).

α1 Receptors respond to epinephrine more than norepinephrine, resulting in vascular smooth muscle contraction or vasoconstriction. α1 Receptors also result in increased sphincter tone and decreased motility of the gastrointestinal track, increased glycogenolysis in the liver, and increased sweating of the skin (4).

α2 Receptors respond to norepinephrine more than epinephrine, resulting in vascular smooth muscle contraction (vasoconstriction). α2 Receptors also cause increased sphincter tone and decreased motility of the gastrointestinal tract, and decreased insulin and glucagon release (4).

β1 Receptors respond equally to epinephrine and norepinephrine. Activation of the β1 receptors causes increased contraction strength of the heart, increased heart rate, increased renin release by the kidney, and increased lipolysis (4).

β2 Receptors respond to epinephrine much greater than norepinephrine. β2 Receptor activation causes vascular smooth muscle (vasodilation), increased renin release by the kidney, increased sphincter tone and decreased motility of the gastrointestinal tract, increased insulin and glucagon release by the pancreas, increased glycogenolysis and gluconeogenesis by the liver, and bronchiolar dilation (4).

β3 Receptor activation causes increased lipolysis by the adipose tissue (4).

Vasoactive Peptides

Peptides are a group of amino acids connected by an amide or peptide bond. They are similar to, but smaller than, proteins. They are responsible for a wide variety of functions, many of which are not yet understood. Peptides are important in cell-to-cell communication. Several peptides possess vaso-constriction properties. These include vasopressin, angiotensin II, endothelins, urotensin, and neuropeptide Y.

Vasopressin or antidiuretic hormone (ADH) is important in short-term regulation of arterial pressure. It is secreted by the posterior pituitary glands. It increases peripheral resistance when infused in low doses. Several analogues of vasopressin have been synthesized and used for their vasoconstrictive properties. Vasopressin and its analogues activate a variety of receptors. Important to this discussion, vasopressin and its analogues activate the Vla receptors, which causes release of phospholipase C, which in turn causes vasoconstriction (5).

Several vasoactive peptides are used as vasoconstrictors in local anesthetic solutions available outside of the United States.

VASOACTIVE DRUGS USED IN DERMATOLOGIC SURGERY

Epinephrine

The most important vasoconstrictor used for vasoconstriction in local anesthetics is epinephrine. The history of epinephrine is very interesting. Oliver and Schafer first demonstrated the pressor effect of extracts derived from the adrenal gland in 1895 (6). John Jacob Abel first isolated a benzoyl derivative (7) of epinephrine from the adrenal gland in 1897 and named it *epinephrine,* meaning from above (epi) the kidney (nephros) (8). Epinephrine was first *crystallized* by Jokichi Takamine in 1901. Takamine was a chemist living in New York, who had ties with Parke-Davis Company when in 1900 he visited Dr. Abel's laboratory at Johns Hopkins. Takamine returned to his own laboratory and produced crystalline material from the adrenal, later shown to be a mixture of epinephrine and norepinephrine. A patent was applied for and the trademark "Adrenalin" was granted in 1901. Adrenaline was marketed by Parke-Davis and soon became a very popular medical and recreational drug. As there was scandal associated with adrenaline, "epinephrine" became the term most commonly used in the United States for this product (7). Epinephrine remains the preferred term in the United States, while adrenaline is used commonly elsewhere. Stolz and Dakin first artificially synthesized epinephrine in 1904. In 1903, Braun reported the use of epinephrine mixed with cocaine to reduce bleeding during surgery, and described such use as similar to a "chemical tourniquet." Commercial mixtures of epinephrine with lidocaine first became available in 1948 (9).

Chemistry (10)

Chemical formula: $C_9H_{13}NO_3$
Chemical name: (*R*)-1-(3,4-Dihydroxyphenyl) –2-(methyl-amino) ethanol
Molecular weight: 183.2
Solubility: Freely soluble in solutions of mineral acid and alkalis; slightly
  soluble in water but forms water-soluble salts with acid

Description: White or creamy white, odorless, crystalline powder; slightly bitter

Source: May be extracted or synthesized

Pharmacology

Epinephrine is a sympathomimetic agent with pronounced effects on $\alpha1$-, $\alpha2$-, and $\beta2$-adrenergic receptors. In low concentrations, epinephrine primarily causes $\beta2$ activation, which activates adenylcyclase, which in turn results in vasodilation in the muscles (11). In higher concentrations, epinephrine also activates the $\alpha1$ and 2 receptors, which activates G proteins and phospholipase C, which in turn causes vasoconstriction of the skin and viscera (11). A summary of the effects of epinephrine is outlined in Table 1.

Pharmacokinetics

Oral administration of epinephrine does not achieve significant blood levels of epinephrine because it is rapidly oxidized and conjugated by the intestine and liver. If given by subcutaneous injection where $\alpha1$-receptor activation causes vasoconstriction, epinephrine release is slow. With administration of epinephrine in the muscle, where $\beta2$-receptor activation causes vasodilation, there is rapid absorption of epinephrine into the blood stream (10).

The plasma half-life of epinephrine is very short (3–10 minutes). It is rapidly taken up by the neurons, oxidized in the liver and neuronal tissues, methylated by catechol-O-methyltransferase, and oxidized by monoamine oxidase (MAO). From 70–95% of metabolized epinephrine may be excreted in the urine after an IV dose (10).

Pharmaceuticals

Epinephrine is the most common vasoconstrictor used in local anesthetics. It is premixed with local anesthetics, usually in a 1:100,000 (0.01 mg/mL) or 1:200,000 dilution (0.005 mg/mL). Dilution of stock epinephrine solution is strongly discouraged, as improper dilutions may be responsible for old reports of necrosis of fingers and toes.

Epinephrine is sensitive to air and light. It should be stored protected from light and remains stable for longer if kept at cool temperatures. It should be discarded if it degrades to a pink- to brown-colored solution (12). Epinephrine is very unstable at pHs higher than 5.5 (12), and is therefore acidified to prolong shelf life.

Local anesthetics with epinephrine have been neutralized with sodium bicarbonate to reduce the pain of infiltration, but should either be neutralized immediately before injection or mixed under sterile hood, labeled, kept cool, and protected from light. Buffered epinephrine degrades to about 90% of its original dosage under these conditions in about two weeks (13).

Heat sterilizing of dental cartridges can be done with relatively small loss of epinephrine with autoclaving (14).

Therapeutic Use

Epinephrine is the most commonly used vasoconstrictor mixed with local anesthetics. Epinephrine dilutions of 1:80,000 to 1:200,000 are most commonly used (10). Although studies comparing epinephrine dilutions of 1:200,000 to 1:400,000 showed that both were effective in providing hemostasis, dilutions of 1:800,000 were significantly less effective (15).

The dosage of epinephrine used with local anesthetics is somewhat unclear. The maximum dosage of epinephrine varies greatly, depending on the patient's age, weight, and route of administration, site of injection, procedure performed, and medical condition of the patient. As the total safe dose for an individual person can be so variable, it is best to always use the minimum amount possible. For adults and adolescents, a usual recommended maximum subcutaneous dose is 0.01 mg/kg to a maximum of 0.3 to 0.5 mg of epinephrine (60 to 100 mL of a solution containing epinephrine 1:200,000) (16). Thus, the dose limitation of lidocaine (1%) with epinephrine (1:200,000) is usually the dose limitation of the lidocaine.

The usual maximum pediatric dose of epinephrine given subcutaneously is 0.01 mg/kg up to a maximum of 0.03 mg/dose (16). Here also the dose limitation of lidocaine (1%) with epinephrine (1:200,000) is usually the dose limitation of the lidocaine.

Epinephrine is used in nonstandard doses in tumescent anesthesia. Large volume anesthesia was introduced by Klein in 1982, initially being used for liposuction. Its use then expanded into other cosmetic and skin surgeries. Epinephrine provides hemostatis and also slows the absorption of the local anesthetics. There is little information regarding the levels of epinephrine in tumescent anesthesia, as most studies measured the blood levels of lidocaine. One study measured the blood levels of lidocaine and epinephrine at 3, 12, and 23 hours and large volume anesthesia. The mean dose of epinephrine after tumescent liposuction when used concurrently with subcutaneous lidocaine and epinephrine for other aesthetic procedures with other aesthetic surgery was 4.96 mg, with a range of 2.2 to 7.0 mg. Peak blood levels of epinephrine were measured at three hours, with the serum epinephrine levels ranging from less than 200 to more than 600 pg/mL. The peak blood level of epinephrine at three hours was approximately three to five times the estimated upper limits of normal. The majority of patients returned to normal blood levels by 12 hours. Blood levels of epinephrine were not drawn sooner than three hours after injection, although the author surmised that the peak blood level actually occurred within 30 minutes of injection (17). A review of over 500 patients in which tumescent anesthesia was used for phlebectomy while using epinephrine (1:100,000) mixed with an anesthesia with total volumes from 175 to 550 cc resulted in no epinephrine-related complications (17).

Klein cautions that epinephrine may cause tachycardia, tremors, and anxiety in patients undergoing tumescent anesthesia, and should be used with caution in patients taking pseudoephedrine for nasal decongestion or those taking dietary supplements containing ephedrine-like compounds. Clonidine, 0.1 mg preoperatively, can be used in patients without bradycardia or hypotension to reduce the incidence of tachycardia in tumescent anesthesia (18). Klein also indicates that the amount of epinephrine per liter used in tumescent anesthesia depends on the location injected. Epinephrine 1 mg/L can be used in fibrous areas of fat such as the upper abdomen, back, and flank, while epinephrine 0.65 mg/L is used in other areas (18).

Epinephrine is also used in topical anesthetics. Compounded formulas of tetracaine/epinephrine/cocaine (TEC or TAC) or tetracaine/lidocaine/epinephrine (TLE or LET) provide effective topical anesthesia for minor dermal procedures (19). LET has been shown to be as effective as TAC (20), without the abuse potential, record keeping hassle, and storage requirements associated with products containing cocaine.

Contraindication

Contraindications to epinephrine include hypersensitivity to the epinephrine, severe hypertension, hyperthyroidism, severe ischemic heart disease, and narrow-angle glaucoma (19).

Precautions (19)

Precautions for use of epinephrine include, but are not limited to, diabetes ($\alpha 2$-receptor suppression of insulin release may cause hyperglycemia) (10), cardiovascular disease and use with drugs that may sensitize the heart to arrhythmias (e.g., digoxin, quinidine), and hypertension. Epinephrine should be injected with caution in patients with severe peripheral vascular disease as intense vasoconstriction may result in tissue necrosis.

The use of epinephrine has long been cautioned against or contraindicated in fingers, toes, penis, or end organs. This dogma has been recently reevaluated by several authors. A comprehensive review of the literature by Denkler from 1880 to 2000 revealed a total of 17 cases of digital gangrene after anesthetic blocks in which unknown concentrations of epinephrine were manually diluted. None of these cases occurred after the introduction of commercially mixed lidocaine and epinephrine in 1948, and may be related to incorrect dilution (9). Denkler provides specific recommendations with regard to use of anesthetics containing epinephrine in the digits. Infiltration of phentolamine has been used for accidental injection of epinephrine (1:1000) into the finger (see section on "Phentolamine").

Adverse Reactions

Severe adverse reactions to epinephrine have included, but are not limited to, cardiac arrhythmias, cerebral hemorrhage, pulmonary edema, hypertensive crisis, seizures, and death (10).

Common adverse reactions include anxiety, dyspnea, restlessness, palpitations, tachycardia, tremors, weakness, dizziness, headache, and coldness of the extremities. There may be stinging or redness of the eyes with epinephrine eyedrops (10).

High-Risk Groups

Neonates: Little documentation

Breast milk: Epinephrine is presumed to be safe, as the oral route cannot reach active levels of epinephrine.

Children: Use in children requires that the body weight is known, and total does calculated.

Pregnant women: High doses have been shown to cause uterine artery spasm and decreased placental perfusion (21), although it has been shown that the levels of endogenous epinephrine are much higher from emotional stress than from local anesthetics (22). Epinephrine has been associated with slightly increased congenital malformations (10).

Pregnancy category: C

Elderly: The elderly are more sensitive to effects of epinephrine and doses should be reduced accordingly (10).

Drug Interactions

Monoamine oxidase inhibitors (MAOIs) may interact with epinephrine to produce severe hypertension. MAO is one of the enzymes that metabolize epinephrine. Reduced epinephrine metabolism due to MAO inhibitors results in prolonged adrenergic receptor stimulation (19).

Tricyclic antidepressants usage has resulted in a two- to fourfold increase in pressor response to epinephrine given by IV infusion (10); however, the local use of epinephrine (local anesthesia) in dilutions of 1:100,000 or less is less likely to precipitate significant hemodynamic changes (23).

Cyclopropane or halogenated hydrocarbon anesthetic increases the risk of epinephrine-induced arrhythmias and pulmonary edema (10).

β-blocking agents, as expected, block the β-receptor activity of epinephrine, resulting in unopposed α-receptor activity (24). This may result in severe hypertension and reflex bradycardia (10). A study of 114 patients given from 1 to 9 mL of lidocaine with epinephrine (1:100,000) resulted in no adverse reactions and no significant changes in blood pressure (25). They concluded that discontinuation of β-blockers is not routinely necessary if small amounts of epinephrine are to be used in dermatologic surgery.

Drug Incompatibilities

Sodium bicarbonate 5% with epinephrine 4 mg/mL results in rapid decomposition, with 58% loss of epinephrine immediately after mixing (12).

Phenylephrine Hydrochloride

Phenylephrine is essentially a pure α stimulator, as opposed to epinephrine, which also has β-receptor activity (26). It has limited use as a topical vasoconstrictor as it is a less effective vasoconstrictor than epinephrine.

Chemistry (10)

Chemical formula: $C(9)H(13)NO(2)HCl$
Chemical name: (*R*)-3-Hydroxy-α [(methylamino)methyl]benzene
   methanol
Molecular weight: 203.7
Solubility: Soluble in water (1:2) and in alcohol
Description: Odorless, bitter tasting, white crystalline powder
Source: Prepared by chemical synthesis

Pharmacology

Phenylephrine is a relatively selective agonist of $\alpha 1$ receptors resulting in vasoconstriction, although it may have a slight, weak agonist effect on $\alpha 2$ and β receptors. The effect of $\alpha 1$ receptors is greater on the venous vessels than the arteriolar vessels (10). There is an increase in blood pressure and reflex bradycardia; however, it has very little direct effect on the heart or its pacemaker. The incidence of cardiac arrhythmia is extremely low (26). Blood flow to the kidneys, skin, skeletal muscles, and splanchnic blood vessels is reduced, and there are no significant CNS effects (10). Phenylephrine is, however, a less effective vasoconstrictor in local anesthetics than epinephrine (26).

Pharmacokinetics

Phenylephrine is irregularly absorbed orally, with systemic availability being about 40%. Peak concentrations are at one to two hours with plasma half-life of two to three hours. Phenylephrine does not seem to cross to the placenta, and excretion in breast milk is not documented (10).

   Phenylephrine taken orally is metabolized largely in the intestine by sulfate conjugation, and the absorbed phenylephrine is metabolized by oxidative deamination by MAOIs in the liver (10). The unchanged phenylephrine (16.6%) and phenylephrine metabolites are then excreted in the urine.

Pharmaceuticals

Phenylephrine is available as a parenteral solution (1 mL of 1% solution), a nasal decongestant (0.1–5%) and mydriatic agent in the eyes (2.5–10%), and as oral decongestants (10). Outside of the United States, phenylephrine is used as a topical vasoconstrictor in rectal ointments, which consist of betamethasone valerate (0.05%), lidocaine (2.5%), and phenylephrine HCl (0.1%).

Phenylephrine is also used as a vasoconstrictor for treatment of superficial lacerations (see the next section).

Phenylephrine products should be protected from light, and discarded if cloudy.

Therapeutic Uses

Phenylephrine is used frequently for treatment of cardiopulmonary resuscitation and hypotension (titrated up to 10 mg), as a topical vasoconstrictor and decongestant for the nose and rectal mucosa, as a mydriatic agent in the eyes, and as a poorly absorbed oral decongestant (up to 40 mg/day) (10). It has also been used to treat priapism. Phenylephrine has been used with local anesthetics or for nerve blocks and spinal anesthesia, although there is little information regarding this use.

Phenylephrine as a vasoconstrictor is used in several compounded topical anesthetic agents used for repair of superficial lacerations. A comparison of Prilophen [prilocaine (3.56%), phenylephrine (0.10%)] and Bupiviphen [bupivacaine (0.67%), phenylephrine (0.10%)] in which a gauze was saturated with 3-mL solution and held over the laceration for 20 minutes demonstrated that Prilophen was as effective as TAC (tetracaine 1%, adrenaline 1:4000, cocaine 4%) in providing hemostasis and topical anesthesia (27). Phenylephrine has also been compounded by mixing 1-mL phenylephrine (1%) in 4-mL lidocaine (4%) and used as a nasal mucosal anesthetic and vasoconstrictor instead of topical cocaine (28). There is no consensus as to total dose/kg, although the initial dose recommended for control of nasal bleeding following surgery should not exceed 0.5 mg (4 drops of a 0.25% nasal solution) (29).

Contraindications

Concurrent use of MAOIs with phenylephrine is contraindicated (10).

Precautions

Precautions to the use of phenylephrine include, but are not limited to, patients on tricyclic antidepressants, patients with hypertension, unstable angina or recent myocardial infarction, or hyperthyroidism (10).

Because of the potential for systemic absorption, serious cardiovascular and hemodynamic responses must be considered. One drop of the 10% ophthalmic solution may contain between 3.5 to 6.7 mg of phenylephrine, which can be rapidly absorbed. The usual upper limit of dosing for IV use is 1.5 mg (30).

Adverse Effects

Adverse side effects of phenylephrine include, but are not limited to, severe hypertension, headache, vomiting, and profound reflex bradycardia, even after topical application. Tissue necrosis may occur if injected subcutaneously (10).

High-Risk Groups

Neonates: Should not exceed 2.5% topical solutions of phenylephrine.

Breast milk: Does not seem to cross to the placenta, and excretion in breast milk is not documented (10).

Children: Should not exceed 2.5% topical solutions of phenylephrine.

Pregnant women: There is potential for uterine contraction and vasoconstriction. Phenylephrine is best avoided during pregnancy. There is no evidence of mutagenic potential and very little crosses the placenta. No reported carcinogenicity (10).

Pregnancy category: C (19).

Elderly: No greater than 2.5% solutions for topical application preferred (10).

Drug Interaction

Hypertension may occur when given with MAOIs and tricyclic antidepressants, ganglion-blocking agents, adrenergic-blocking drugs, rauwolfia alkaloids, and methyldopa (10).

Norepinephrine

Norepinephrine is a naturally occurring, powerful vasoconstrictor; however, it has significant adverse side effects, and therefore not commonly used as a vasoconstrictor in local anesthetics.

Chemistry (10)

Chemical formula: $C(8)H(11)NO(3)H(6)O(6)H(2)O$

Chemical name: (*R*)-4-(2-Amino-1-hydroxyethyl)-1,2-benzenediol hydrogen tartarate

Molecular weight: 337.3

Solubility: Soluble in water (1:2.5)

Description: Odorless, white or faint gray crystalline powder with bitter taste

Source: Extracted from natural sources or synthesized

Pharmacology

Norepinephrine is an agonist of $\alpha 1$ and $\beta 1$ receptors. It primarily affects the $\alpha 1$ receptors, causing intense vasoconstriction. Blood flow through the skeletal muscles is decreased. The limited $\beta 1$ activation causes increased cardiac contractility, increase in heart rate, and enhanced cardiac conduction (19). Norepinephrine is 10 times less active in producing metabolic responses than epinephrine (10), and is about 4 times less vasoconstrictive than epinephrine. As there is less vasoconstriction compared with epinephrine, the norepinephrine is absorbed more rapidly than epinephrine, and with greater consequences. The absence of $\beta 2$ response and unopposed $\alpha 1$ and $\beta 1$ stimulation result in pronounced hypertension and risk of toxicity (11).

Pharmacokinetics

Norepinephrine is rapidly and extensively metabolized in the gut and liver. It is slowly absorbed from subcutaneous sites because of its vasoconstrictive effect. Bioavailability by subcutaneous injection and oral ingestion is poor (19). The half-life of norepinephrine is short—from 0.6 to 2.9 minutes. Norepinephrine is metabolized primarily in liver by cathechol-*O*-methyltransferase and MAO (19), and largely excreted in urine (10).

Norepinephrine darkens on exposure to air and light, and turns brown in alkaline or neutral solution. It is incompatible with alkaline solutions, iron salts, and oxidizing agents.

Pharmaceutics

Norepinephrine is available mixed with local anesthetics intended primarily for dental use. Premixed dental cartridges contain propoxycaine hydrochloride (7.2 mg/1.8 mL), procaine (36 mg/1.8 mL), and norepinephrine (0.12 mg/mL) (19). Outside of the United States, lidocaine or carbocaine with norepinephrine is available for dental anesthesia (31).

Products containing norepinephrine should be stored below 25°C, protected from light, and should be discarded if precipitate forms (12).

Therapeutic Use

The most common use of norepinephrine is for parenteral treatment of hypotension. It is also used for cardiac stimulation, treatment of shock, GI bleeding, and glaucoma to stimulate abortions and as an adjunct to tetracaine in spinal anesthesia (32). As an adjuvant in local anesthesia, norepinephrine has been used in concentrations of 1:80,000 (10). The use of norepinephrine has been forbidden in some countries because severe hypertension has been associated with its use (33).

Contraindications

Norepinephrine is contraindicated in blood volume deficit (10), severe hypertension, severe hyperthyroidism, severe ischemic heart disease, and recent history of myocardial infarction.

Precautions

Norepinephrine should be used with caution in patients with vascular thrombosis, in conjunction with cyclopropane and halothane anesthesia, under conditions of profound hypoxia or hypercarbia, in conjunction with MAOI or tricyclic antidepressants, and in patients with sulfite allergy.

Adverse Reactions

Severe adverse reactions associated with norepinephrine usage have included, but are not limited to, platelet aggregation, hypertension, cerebral hemorrhage, pulmonary edema, nephrotoxicity, reflex bradycardia, arrhythmias, angina, palpitations, cardiac arrest, and sudden death (19).

Adverse skin reactions have included tissue necrosis, sloughing, and gangrene (19). Sloughing and necrosis have occurred around parenteral norepinephrine injection sites along with gangrene of extremities (10). Extravasation of norepinephrine should be treated immediately with infiltration with phentolamine.

In a review of adverse reactions after having received a local anesthetic with norepinephrine (1:25,000), 15 patients reported severe reactions, including severe headaches, chest tightness, and subarachnoid hemorrhage (19).

High-Risk Groups

Neonates: The effects of norepinephrine are not well documented (10).
Breast milk: The effect of norepinephrine on breast milk is unknown (19). Norepinephrine levels do not achieve active levels after oral administration, and therefore should not present any problem to infants.
Children: The risks of norepinephrine are the same as with adults (10).
Pregnant women: Norepinephrine should be avoided in pregnancy. Contractile action may lead to fetal asphyxia in late pregnancy (10). Pregnancy category: C
Elderly: The elderly are particularly susceptible to effects of norepinephrine (10).

Drug Interactions

Norepinephrine should be used with great caution in association with MAOIs and tricyclic antidepressants, as these drugs interfere with the metabolism of norepinephrine, resulting in severe hypertension, cardiac arrhythmias, and tachycardia. Norepinephrine is less likely than epinephrine to produce arrhythmias when used with halogenated anesthetic agents, but must be used with great caution (10). Norepinephrine should also be used with caution with adrenergic blocking agents, methyldopa, and digoxin (10).

Levonordefrin (Corbadrine)

Levonordefrin is a norepinephrine derivative and a vasoconstrictor that is used primarily in dentistry. It has the advantage of being much more stable than epinephrine.

Chemistry (31)

Chemical formula: C(9)H(13)NO(2)
Chemical name: (–)-Amino-1-(3,4-dihydroxyphenyl)propan-1-ol
Molecular weight: 183.2
Solubility: Practically insoluble in water, slightly soluble in alcohol, and freely soluble in aqueous solution of mineral acids
Description: White to buff-colored, odorless crystalline solid
Source: Synthetic (11)

Pharmacology

Levonordefrin is an adrenergic vasoconstrictor similar to that of norepinephrine, although much weaker. Ten times the dose of levonordefrin is required to produce a similar effect as to that of norepinephrine (11).

Pharmacokinetics

Levonordefrin is more slowly metabolized than norepinephrine because the presence of a methyl group prevents the more rapid degradation of the levonordefrin by MAO (11).

Pharmaceutics

There is limited use of levonordefrin in the United States. The only present premixed source is that of dental cartridges of mepivacaine (2%) mixed with levonordefrin (0.05 mg/mL) (19). Outside of the United States, levonordefrin is also mixed with procaine and tetracaine hydrochlorides, and propoxycaine and procaine hydrochlorides (19).

Levonordefrin dilutions of 1:20,000 have been used in combination with local anesthetics (31).

Therapeutic Use

Levonordefrin is used primarily as a vasoconstrictor in anesthetics used for dentistry (34).

Contraindications

Contraindication include allergy to sulfites, which is used to preserve levonordefrin.

Precautions

Levonordefrin should be used with great caution in patients with hypertension, arteriosclerotic heart disease, cerebral vascular insufficiency, hyperthyroidism, and diabetes (34).

Adverse Reactions

Adverse reactions to levonordefrin include, but are not limited to, chest pain, hypertension, restlessness, rapid heart rate, nervousness, dizziness, blurred vision, and possible respiratory arrest and cardiovascular reactions (34).

High-Risk Groups

Neonates: It is not known if levonordefrin is secreted in mother's milk (35).
Children: Data not available.
Pregnant women: There is very limited information on use in pregnancy; however, the frequency of congenital abnormalities was no greater in a small number of patients (26) in the first four months of pregnancy than in those not exposed (36).
Pregnancy category: C (35)
Elderly: Data not available.

Drug Interactions

Severe hypertension may be precipitated by concomitant use of MOAIs or tricyclic antidepressants (35).

Ornipressin (POR-8)

Ornipressin is a synthetic derivative of vasopressin and has been used to control bleeding during surgery. It was once thought that it might become the vasoconstrictor of choice for hemostasis in the operative field (37). However, its powerful coronary vasoconstrictor effects, along with reports of severe complications, have led to its near abandonment in surgical hemostasis (11).

Chemistry (31)

Chemical formula: $C(45)H(63)N(13)O(12)S(2)$
Chemical name: [8-Ornithine]-vasopressin

Molecular weight: 1042.2
Description: Clear acidic solution (pH 3.7) (37)
Source: Synthetic derivative of vasopressin

Pharmacology

Ornipressin is a synthetic derivative of vasopressin. It is a strong vasoconstrictor with only weak antidiuretic properties (37).

Binding of ornipressin to the V_{1a} receptors results in activation of G_s protein, phospholipase C activation, and vasoconstriction. Most studies have shown that ornipressin is similar in effect to adrenaline with regard to vaso-constriction, with fewer side effects (37).

Pharmacokinetics

The onset of activity of ornipressin occurs within three minutes with tissue infiltration (37). Topical application of ornipressin to debrided areas produces hemostasis within 20 seconds (38). The duration of action of ornipressin is about 45 to 120 minutes (37). Ornipressin is metabolized in the liver and kidneys.

Pharmaceutics

Ornipressin is available outside of the United States in ampules of 5 IU/mL. There is little guideline as to the dosage to be used; however, the manufacturer recommends that ornipressin be administered in concentrations of 5 IU diluted in 30 mL of normal saline (0.17 IU/mL) (37).

Therapeutic Use

The local vasoconstrictor property of ornipressin is almost equivalent to that of epinephrine. Ornipressin solutions have been used with and without local anesthetics to control bleeding in burn treatment, gynecologic procedures, scalp infiltration for neurosurgery procedures, and in prostatic surgery (37). Intrave-nous ornipressin has also been used to treat esophageal varices (31).

For hemostasis, solutions containing up to 5 U of ornipressin in 20 to 60 mL of 0.9% sodium chloride are infiltrated into the area involved (31). There is wide variation in amounts of ornipressin actually used, although doses of 0.01 IU/mL were adequate in most cases. The maximum total dose of ornipressin is 5 IU (37). High doses or ornipressin may cause vasodilation (39).

Contraindications

Contraindications to use of ornipressin include coronary heart disease, severe hypertension, toxemia of pregnancy, advanced arteriosclerosis, and epilepsy (2).

Precautions

Ornipressin must be used with caution in patients with hypertension and severe heart disease. Few other recommendations are available.

Adverse Reactions

The use of ornipressin has been associated with, but not limited to, acute pulmonary edema (31). There are cases in which patients have had "immeasurable" blood pressure after its use (2). An increase in arterial pressure of 0–25% in response to infiltration or infusion of ornipressin has been seen (37). Arrhythmias have also been reported with use of ornipressin (40).

High-Risk Groups

Neonates: No data found.
Children: No data found.
Pregnant women: There is no evidence of teratogenicity or mutagenicity in animal studies; however, vasopressor agents may reduce blood flow to the pregnant uterus.
Elderly: No data found.

Drug Interactions

No data was found.

Felypressin (Octapressin)

Felypressin is a synthetic analog of the antidiuretic hormone, vasopressin. It produces vasoconstriction by directly stimulating vascular smooth muscle (26). Information regarding felypressin is very sparse.

Chemistry (31)

Chemical formula: $C(46)H(65)N(13)O(11)S(2)$
Chemical name: [2-Phenylalanine, 8-lysine]vasopressin
Molecular weight: 1040.2
Source: Synthetic analog of the antidiuretic hormone, vasopressin

Pharmacology

Felypressin is similar in pharmacologic activity to vasopressin. It causes vasoconstriction through activation of the V1a receptors (5), although it has a vasoconstricting ability that is five times that of vasopressin (41). V1a receptor activation is also responsible for coronary vasoconstriction (42). Animal studies have shown a 49% reduction of coronary blood flow during infusion of felypressin (41).

Pharmacokinetics

There is little information regarding the pharmacokinetics of felypressin; however, the metabolism would be similar to that of vasopressin in which there is reduction of the disulfide bond and peptide cleavage in the kidney and the liver (43).

Pharmaceutics

Felypressin is available outside of the United States as premixed dental anesthetic, usually in combination with prilocaine (31). The standard concentration of felypressin is 0.03 IU/mL.

Therapeutic Use

Felypressin is used primarily in combination with prilocaine for dental anesthesia. The usual dosage of prilocaine (3%) felypressin (0.03 IU/mL) in a normal adult is 1 to 5 mL, with a maximum dose of 10 mL (44). One study has showed a maximum safe amount of the felypressin in a patient with essential hypertension as being 0.18 IU or 6 mL of the previously mentioned anesthetic mixture (45). Felypressin is used as a substitute vasoconstrictor for epinephrine. It was initially thought not to cause vasoconstriction of the coronary vessels (11). Animal studies, however, show significant coronary vasoconstriction (41).

Contraindications and Precautions

Felypressin is contraindicated if there is known hypersensitivity to its ingredients. Although other contraindications are not clearly defined, felypressin is closely related to vasopressin and lypressin, and contraindications may be similar to these products.

Adverse Reactions

There is little data on the side effects of felypressin.

High-Risk Groups

Neonates: Not available.
Children: Not available.
Pregnant women: Felypressin may interfere with the tonicity of the
uterus resulting in compromised fetal circulation (31).
Elderly: Not available.

Drug Interactions

Drug interactions with felypressin are not available.

Cocaine

Cocaine was first used as an anesthetic in modern medicine in 1885 when Carl found it effective in anesthetizing the cornea. Its use as a local anesthetic spread rapidly. The great benefit of cocaine was that it was not only a good anesthetic, but it was also an excellent vasoconstrictor. Its toxicity and potential for abuse have limited its usefulness.

Chemistry

Chemical name: 2-β-carbomethoxy-3-β-benzoxy tropane (19)
Molecular weight: 303.365
Solubility: Soluble in water and freely soluble in alcohol (46)
Description: An ester-type local anesthetic, available as a hydrochloride
   salt, which is a colorless or white crystalline powder (46)
Source: Derived from the leaves of *Erythroxylon coca* and the only
   naturally occurring anesthetic

Pharmacology

Following topical application, cocaine blocks the induction and conduction of nerve impulses, which causes the anesthetic effect (47).

Cocaine also has important vasoconstrictive properties. It blocks norepinephrine uptake at the adrenergic nerve receptor sites, which results in the increased concentration of norepinephrine at the receptor sites, which in turn results in vasoconstriction (48). Cocaine may also promote the release of norepinephrine (47).

Pharmacokinetics

Cocaine is well absorbed from mucous membranes and the GI tract, with increased absorption if inflammation is present. The onset of anesthetic activity occurs approximately 1 minute after topical application of cocaine, with the duration of action lasting 20 to 40 minutes. The peak serum level occurs 20 to 60 minutes after intranasal use, with the half-life being approximately 75 minutes (19).

Cocaine is rapidly hydrolyzed by serum cholinesterase in the blood, and undergoes N-demethylation in the liver (49). The metabolites are largely excreted in the urine (85–90%), with 1% to 20% being excreted unchanged (50).

Pharmaceutics

Cocaine hydrochloride is available as crystal flakes, tablets for formulation, and topical and viscous solutions [40 mg/mL (4%) and 100 mg/mL (10%)] (19). The cocaine is reformulated for the particular application.

Cocaine HCl should be stored in light-resistant containers at 15°C to 30°C (46). Cocaine is stable at a pH of 5 or lower. A change in the pH may result in loss of stability (19).

Therapeutic Use

Cocaine is used for topical anesthesia when vasoconstriction of mucous membranes is useful, such as during procedures in the mouth, larynx, and nasal cavities. It is generally not used in ocular mucosa because of potential toxicity (19).

For mucosal anesthesia, solutions of 1–10% cocaine are used, although concentrations greater than 4% are not generally recommended because of difficulty in controlling the dosage, and the risk of complications (16). A dose of 1 mg/kg or 150 to 200 mg should generally not be exceeded (19). A maximum dose of 1 mg/kg has been recommended to reduce the risk of toxicity. In all cases, the lowest possible doses should be used for topical application.

TAC, a solution of tetracaine (0.5%), epinephrine (1:2000), and cocaine (11.8%), has frequently been used as a topically anesthetic and hemostatic for treatment of small lacerations, especially in children (51). The recommended dose is 2 to 5 mL in lacerations up to 5 cm. Some have recommended a dose of 1 mL/cm of laceration. TAC solution should be applied as a *single* dose, with the smallest volume possible. The application will be most effective if left in place for 30 to 40 minutes before a procedure (51). Half-strength TAC has also been used successfully because of the risk of toxic effects of cocaine. The plasma level of cocaine 30 minutes after intranasal administration of 1.5 mg/kg (10% solution) was 331 ng/mL (52), whereas following topical application of 3 mL of standard TAC solution (tetracaine 0.5%, epinephrine 0.05%, cocaine 11.9%) for 15 minutes to a laceration in children, the median concentrations was 1 to 2 ng/mL (53).

Cocaine gel formulations can also be used as an alternative to TAC solution to reduce the cocaine requirement. Methylcellulose powder (0.15 grams) is mixed with 1.5mL of a standard cocaine-adrenaline solution (cocaine 11.8%, adrenaline 1:2000). An average of 0.35 mL of the gel is required per laceration (54). A variety of other mixtures of local anesthetics and vasoconstrictors other than cocaine have been effectively used (see sec. "Vasoconstrictors in Topical Mixtures").

Contraindications

Cocaine is contraindicated in patients with known hypersensitivity to cocaine, severe cardiovascular disease, severe cerebrovascular disease, and uncontrolled hypertension.

Precautions

Cocaine should be used with caution in patients with atypical cholinesterase and/or succinylcholine sensitivity (52). Cocaine is not recommended for direct instillation into the eyes. It should be used with caution in areas of sepsis and in severely traumatized mucosa (19).

Adverse Reactions

Side effects of cocaine are due largely to the sympathetic activity. The fatal dose of cocaine is reported to be 1.2 g; however, there is great patient variability. Adverse effects are reported with as little as 20 mg (16). The average blood concentration in individuals who died after injection of cocaine averaged 0.03 to 0.3 mg/dL (55). Cocaine is absorbed very rapidly through the mucosal membranes, reaching peak levels in 5 minutes (16). Toxic reactions may progress through three stages—early stimulation, advanced stimulation, and eventually depression (16).

Side effects include, but are not limited to, severe hypertension, cardiac arrhythmias, CNS hemorrhage, congestive heart failure, convulsions, excitement, and nervousness (16).

Case reports of topical cocaine are instructive. A report of intranasal instillation of 2 drops of 4% cocaine solution (0.6 to 0.7 mg/kg) in an 11-week-old infant resulted in dramatic toxicity (56). Cardiac ischemia and myocardial infarctions have been reported with therapeutic intranasal use. In nine patients given intranasal cocaine 2 mg/kg (total dose of 100 to 250 mg) reaching serum concentrations between 0.04 to 0.22 mg/L, it was demonstrated that cocaine induces vasoconstriction in both diseased and nondiseased coronary arteries (57). Nitroglycerin alleviated the vasoconstriction. CNS effects, including grand mal seizures, have been reported after application of 2 mL of topical TAC solution (58). Ocular application has resulted in corneal ulcers, clouding, pitting, sloughing, glaucoma, anisocoria, and nystagmus (19).

High-Risk Groups

Neonates: Cocaine readily passes into breast milk (59). Neonates are particularly susceptible to the effects of cocaine as they have slow inactivation of the drug (16).

Children: Because of its toxicity, cocaine is not recommended in children under 6 years, and with caution and reduced doses in children aged 6 years or older (16).

Pregnant women: Cocaine readily crosses the placenta during pregnancy (60). Although multiple fetal abnormalities are found with regular cocaine use during pregnancy, brief exposure in early pregnancy does not appear to affect the outcome of pregnancy (61).

FDA pregnancy category: C

Elderly: Elderly patients are especially sensitive to the effects of cocaine because of reduced metabolism and because of underlying medical conditions, such as cerebrovascular insufficiency or cardiac disease.

Drug/Food Interactions

Cocaine may interact with a wide variety of medications, including general anesthetic agents, tricyclic antidepressants, MAOIs, β-blocking agents, and sympathomimetic agents. Ethanol will also potentiate the effects of cocaine (62). If cocaine is to be used, a complete review of drug interactions should be undertaken.

Ropivacaine Hydrochloride

Ropivacaine hydrochloride is a long-acting amino-amide local anesthetic with a toxicity profile intermediate between bupivacaine and lidocaine. It is the only local anesthetic, other than cocaine, that possesses vasoconstrictive properties.

Chemistry (10)

Chemical formula: $C(17)H(26)N(2)OHClH(2)O$
Chemical name: S-(-)-1-Propyl-2′,6′pipecoloxylidide
Molecular weight: 328.9
Solubility: Soluble in water (1:19)
Description: Odorless, clear liquid
Source: Manufactured in pure S(–) form
Stability: Stable in solution at room temperature and is preservative free

Pharmacology

Ropivacaine acts by reversibly blocking the sodium ion channels in nerve cell membrane (63).

Unlike other local anesthetics other than cocaine, ropivacaine produces significant vasoconstriction in the subcutaneous tissue and skin (63). The effect of ropivacaine given intradermally and subcutaneously is biphasic—when given in small amounts it causes vasoconstriction, but larger volumes may cause vasodilation (10).

Pharmacokinetics

Ropivacaine hydrochloride is well absorbed systemically. It is metabolized in the liver via the cytochrome P450 system (19). The metabolites are excreted primarily through the kidneys (86%) (10). Only a small amount of the unchanged ropivacaine appears in the urine. The onset of action of ropivacaine is 1 to 15 minutes with a duration of 2 to 6 hours, with the half-life after IV doses being about 2 hours (19). There is no evidence of metabolism to the R isomer (toxicity occurs more often with R isomer than with the S isomer (10).

Pharmaceutics

Ropivacaine HCl is available in concentrations of 2 mg/mL, 7.5 mg/mL, 10 mg/mL, in vials of 10 to 30 mL. Ropivacaine is stable in solution at room temperature and should be stored between 15°C and 30°C. Ropivacaine is preservative free (10). Ropivacaine should not be diluted or mixed with other solutions, and precipitation may occur in alkaline solutions (10).

Therapeutic Use

Ropivacaine is used for local and regional anesthesia in surgery, usually as 0.5–1% solutions in doses of 5 to 250 mg (19). It has been used for field blocks, wound infiltration, peripheral nerve block, postoperative epidural infusion, and epidural analgesia in labor (10). It not only possesses anesthetic effect but also has significant vasoconstrictor effects. The degree of vasoconstriction seen with ropivacaine may be equivalent to the vasoconstriction of the skin seen with epinephrine (64).

The maximum recommended dose of ropivacaine HCl is 250 mg in adults. There is no evidence of toxic plasma levels at these levels (10).

Contraindications

Ropivacaine is contraindicated in patients with hypersensitivity to amide-type local anesthetics.

Precautions

Ropivacaine should be used with great caution in patients with severe cardiovascular disease as it is a cardiac depressant. It should also be used with caution in those with severe renal impairment, as toxicity due to reduced clearance may develop (16).

Adverse Reactions

Adverse reactions associated with ropivacaine have included, but are not limited to, hypotension, tachycardia, shivering, urinary retention, nausea and vomiting, and seizures (19). Cardiotoxic and CNS effects appear to be less than that of bupivacaine (19) and are very rare in the absence of IV injection (10). If toxicity develops, CNS toxicity precedes that of cardiotoxicity (10).

High-Risk Groups

Neonates: There are no mutagenic or teratogenic effects found in animal studies given five times the human doses of ropivacaine (10).

Breast milk: The amount of ropivacaine excreted in breast milk is not known in humans; however, the excretion rate is about 4% in rats. It is unlikely that this is a significant amount (10).

Children: There is no dosage recommendation for children less than 12 years of age as there is lack of safety data (16).

Pregnant women: Ropivacaine flows rapidly across the placenta with fetal levels about the same as maternal levels (10). Ropivacaine given during delivery has caused fetal hypotension, bradycardia or tachycardia, and fetal distress (16).

Pregnancy category: B.

Elderly: There are no specific risks associated with use of ropivacaine in the elderly; however, general guidelines for reduction of drug doses should be followed (10).

Drug Interactions

There are no known drug interactions associated with ropivacaine (10). There is the potential for metabolism to be inhibited by other drugs, which are metabolized by cytochrome P450, such as theophylline and imipramine (16). Toxic effects are additive to those of other local anesthetics (16). Smoking might enhance the metabolism of ropivacaine (10).

ANTIDOTE TO ADRENERGIC VASOCONSTRICTORS

Phentolamine (Mesylate)

An important inclusion in the discussion of vasoconstrictors for local anesthetics is a review of antidotes to vasoconstrictors. Phentolamine is an antidote to adrenergic vasoconstrictors. It has been used for treatment of severe vasoconstriction resulting from accidental injection of epinephrine pens into the digits (10).

Pharmacology

Phentolamine is a competitive α antagonist acting on $\alpha1$ and $\alpha2$ receptors, resulting in smooth muscle relaxation, reduced peripheral resistance, and increased venous capacity. It also causes cardiac stimulation (10).

Pharmacokinetics

The onset of phentolamine given IV is immediate (19), with a half-life of 19 minutes when given intravenously (65). It is metabolized extensively in the liver

(66) with about 70% of the metabolites excreted in urine. Only about 10–13% of the unchanged phentolamine is excreted into the urine (10).

Pharmaceutics

Phentolamine is available as a lyophilized powder in vials containing 5 mg. It is reconstituted with 1 ml of sterile water for injection. Phentolamine should be protected from light and stored between 15°C and 30°C. (10).

Therapeutic Use

Phentolamine is usually used for control of blood pressure and is given as an intravenous infusion in 5% dextrose or saline at a rate of 0.2 to 2 mg/min, titrating the dose to the desired blood pressure (10).

As an antidote to local overdose of vasoconstrictors, phentolamine is given by local infusion. Local infiltration can also be used in preventing skin necrosis after extravasation of α-adrenergic agonists. Phentolamine is prepared by diluting 5 to 10 mg in 10-mL 0.9% sterile saline and infiltrating the affected area (10). To be effective, this should occur within 12 hours after the extravasation of the vasoconstrictor (10).

Phentolamine has been used successfully following accidental injection of epinephrine into finger with anaphylactic kits. Treatment consists of infiltrating the area with 0.5% phentolamine mesylate (67).

Contraindications

Contraindication to the use of phentolamine includes hypotension, severe coronary insufficiency or angina, and sensitivity of sulfites, which is used as a preservative (10).

Precautions

Phentolamine should be used with caution in asthmatics, especially in those with sulfite sensitivity, and in patients with gastric or peptic ulcers (10).

Adverse Reactions

Adverse reactions have included hypotension, tachycardia, arrhythmia, headache, angina, myocardial infarction, cerebrospasm, drowsiness, dizziness, weakness, sweating, visual disturbance, hypoglycemia. Severe hypotension and death have occurred in patients with pheochromocytoma (10).

High-Risk Groups

Neonates: It is not known if phentolamine is excreted in breast milk.
Children: Appropriate studies have not been performed (16).

Pregnant women: Pregnant women should avoid phentolamine since
there is insufficient information regarding safety; however,
no mutagenic potential is demonstrated (10).
FDA Pregnancy category: C
Elderly: Increased risk of hypotension (19)

Drug Interactions

Phentolamine should be used carefully in combination with other hypotensive
agents. Phentolamines used along with antipyschotics may cause hypotension
(10). The use of phentolamine may block the α-adrenergic response to epinephrine with possible severe hypotension and tachycardia (16).

VASOCONSTRICTORS AND SPECIAL APPLICATIONS

Vasoconstrictors in Flaps or Grafts

Most information on the use of vasoconstrictors in local anesthetics for flaps and
grafts relates to the use of epinephrine. Studies involving delayed flaps in rats
demonstrate a significant loss of flaps if epinephrine in concentrations of 1:200,000
and 1:400,000 is used (68). The effect of epinephrine in local anesthesia on the
survival of full- and split-thickness skin grafts has also been evaluated in rabbits.
Full-thickness grafts from donor sites infiltrated with plain lidocaine had a mean
survival rate of 85%, whereas donor sites infiltrated with lidocaine with epinephrine
had a mean survival rate of 42% (69). In humans, an evaluation of the impact of
lidocaine with epinephrine versus plain lidocaine for harvesting full-thickness
grafts was evaluated in 72 patients. At one week, 4 of 33 (12%) of the plain
lidocaine group and 16 of 39 (41%) of the lidocaine with epinephrine group had
graft loss, epidermal necrosis, or infection. There was no difference between the
groups, however, in the graft appearance six weeks after surgery (70). Skin-flap
survival has been evaluated in rats in which tumescent anesthesia using lidocaine
and epinephrine (1:100,000, 1:200,000, 1:400,000, or 1:800,000) was used. There
was a significantly higher rate of flap necrosis at seven days in the groups infiltrated
with lidocaine with epinephrine (1:100,000 or 1:200,000) compared with the
groups infiltrated with lidocaine with epinephrine (1:400,000 or 1:800,000) (71). It
has been postulated that the vasoconstrictive properties of epinephrine are prolonged in the graft after it has been removed from the donor site, as the normal
clearance of epinephrine from the graft has been altered (70).

Vasoconstrictors in Topical Mixtures

Various topical anesthetic agents utilizing vasoconstrictors have been useful for
use in superficial lacerations prior to suturing to control bleeding, and to slow
mobilization of the local anesthetic from the laceration site. The original topical

agent (TAC) comprised tetracaine 1%, adrenaline (epinephrine) 1:4000, and cocaine 11.8 % (27). Although this solution is effective, cocaine carries a risk of severe toxic reactions, and has significant abuse and regulatory concerns. Various anesthetics with vasoconstrictors have been evaluated, as follows:

TAC—tetracaine 0.5%, adrenaline 1:2000, cocaine 11.8% (72)
TAC—tetracaine 1%, adrenaline 1:4000, cocaine 11.8% (73).
TAC—tetracaine 1%, adrenaline 1:4000, cocaine 4% (27)
Prilophen—prilocaine 3.56%, phenylephrine 0.10% (27)
Bupivaphen—bupivacaine 0.67%, phenylephrine 0.10% (27)
Tetraphen—tetracaine 1%, phenylephrine 5.0% (74)
Tetralidophen—tetracaine 1%, lidocaine 1%, phenylephrine 2.5% (74)
LET—lidocaine 4%, epinephrine 1:2000, tetracaine 1% (51)

A mixture of lidocaine, epinephrine, and tetracaine (LET) has been shown to be as effective in producing topical anesthesia as TAC (75). As alternatives to TAC are available, they should be considered for topical anesthesia.

Digital Block with Vasoconstrictors

The use of epinephrine for digital blocks has been strictly contraindicated by many sources. This dogma has been recently reevaluated by several authors. A comprehensive review of the literature by Denkler from 1880 to 2000 revealed a total of 17 cases of digital gangrene after anesthetic blocks in which unknown concentrations of epinephrine were manually diluted. The necrosis was probably related to over-distention of the tissues, poor technique, or use of too much epinephrine. None of these cases occurred after the introduction of commercially mixed lidocaine and epinephrine in 1948 and may be related to incorrect dilutions (9).

Blood flow of the digits following digital blocks using lidocaine 2% with epinephrine 1:100,000 was recently evaluated by color Doppler flow imaging in 24 patients. There was a statistically significant reduction of blood flow in all patients within 10 minutes of the digital block. In four patients there was no measurable blood flow at 10 minutes. All patients had return of normal blood flow by 60 to 90 minutes (76). Although the author cautioned against the use of epinephrine in digits in patients with peripheral vascular disease and diabetes, he concluded that lidocaine with epinephrine 1:100,000 is safe in selected patients.

Infiltration of phentolamine has been used for accidental injection of epinephrine (1:1000) into the finger (see section on "Phentolamine").

Vasoconstrictors in Tumescent Anesthesia

The primary vasoconstrictor used for tumescent anesthesia is epinephrine (see sec. "Epinephrine"). Epinephrine provides hemostatis and also slows the absorption of the local anesthetics.

The usefulness of epinephrine in reducing bleeding during tumescent anesthesia has been demonstrated. An evaluation of tumescent anesthesia using lidocaine with epinephrine (1:100,000) for phlebectomy compared with tumescent anesthesia without epinephrine showed a reduced hematoma and complication rate in the group in which epinephrine was used (77).

There is question as to whether tumescent anesthesia and the addition of epinephrine may have a deleterious effect on skin flaps. Ramirez reported superficial flap loss using tumescent anesthesia with epinephrine. This may have been the result of the hydrostatic pressure of the fluid injected combined with the vasoconstrictor effect of epinephrine (78). Animal studies have also shown that tumescent anesthesia with epinephrine 1:100,000 or 1:200,000 are associated with a higher level of flap necrosis (71).

Ropivacaine has been regarded as a major step forward in the field of local anesthesia in Europe (79). Ropivacaine with epinephrine (1:100,000) was evaluated as a slow infusion tumescent agent in 5220 patients, and compared to lidocaine with epinephrine (1:100,000). The patients receiving ropivacaine as the tumescent anesthetic had a prolonged duration of anesthesia when compared with the lidocaine group. There were no minor or major incidents occurring in any of these patients. The author mentions that ropivacaine has vasoconstrictor properties; however, plain ropivacaine without epinephrine was not evaluated in this study, except for blocks of the fingers or penis (79). In another study of 204 children, ropivacaine and prilocaine was infused subcutaneously with no side effects noted (80). There was no clear evaluation of the vasoconstrictor effect. At this point, there are no clear studies evaluating the vasoconstrictive properties of ropivacaine without epinephrine in tumescent anesthesia.

SUMMARY

The use and knowledge of vasoconstrictors has progressed greatly since the first vasoconstrictor, epinephrine, was isolated. Surprisingly, it is still the primary vasoconstrictor used today. Future developments will no doubt provide vasoconstrictors that will be more selective, cause fewer side effects, and react less frequently with other medications.

REFERENCES

1. Katzung BG. Autonomic drugs. In: Katzung BG, ed. Basic and Clinical Pharmacology. New York: McGraw-Hill, 2004.
2. Charkoudian N. Skin blood flow in adult human thermoregulation: how it works, when it does not, and why. Mayo Clin Proc 2003; 78(5):603–612.
3. Klauer K. Adrenal insufficiency and adrenal crisis. In: Alson, R, Talavera, F, Bessen, H, et al., eds. Endocrine and Metabolic. eMedicine from WebMD. Available at: http://www.emedicine.com/emerg/topic16.htm. Accessed August 2004.

4. Hoyer. In: Gore RW. Department of Physiology, University of Arizona, http://human.physiol.arizona.edu.
5. Reid IA. Vasoactive peptides. In: Ganong WF, ed. Review of Medical Physiology. New York: McGraw-Hill, 2004.
6. Hoffman BB. Catecholamines, sympathomimetic drugs, and adrenergic receptor antagonists. In: Hardman JG, Limbird LE, Gilman AG, eds. Goodman & Gilman's The Pharmacological Basis of Therapeutics. New York: McGraw-Hill, 2004: 215–268.
7. Bennett JW. Adrenalin and cherry trees. American Chemical Society. Available at: http://pubs.acs.org/subscribe/journals/mdd/v04/i12/html/12timeline.html#auth. Accessed August 2004.
8. http://www.cartage.org.lb/en/themes/Biographies/MainBiographies/A/AbelJ/1.html. Accessed August 2004.
9. Denkler K. A comprehensive review of epinephrine in the finger: to do or not to do. Plast Reconstr Surg 2001; 108(1):114–124.
10. Dollery C, ed. Therapeutic Drugs. 2nd ed. Edinburgh: Churchill Livingstone, 1999.
11. Madrid C, Bruno C, Vironneau M. Recommendations to use vasoconstrictors in dentistry and oral surgery. Societe Francophone de Medecine Buccale et de Chirurgie Buccale 2003; 9:1–30. Available at: http://www.societechirbuc.com/Recommandations/recommandations_vasoconstricteurs_gb.pdf. Accessed August 2004.
12. Trissel LA. Handbook on Injectable Drugs. 6th ed. Bethesda, MD: American Society of Hospital Pharmacists, 1990.
13. Larson PO, Ragi G, Swandby M, et al. Stability of buffered lidocaine and epinephrine used for local anesthesia. J Dermatol Surg Oncol 1991; 17(5):411–414.
14. Kelly JR, Dalm GW. Stability of epinephrine in dental anesthetic solutions: implications for autoclave sterilization and elevated temperature storage. Mil Med 1985; 150(2):112–114.
15. Dunlevy TM, O'Malley TP, Postma GN. Optimal concentration of epinephrine for vasoconstriction in neck surgery. Laryngoscope 1996; 106(11):1412–1414.
16. USP DI(R) Drug Information for Health Care Professional. Greenwood Village Colorado: Thomson MICROMEDEX, Inc. (Edition expires 2004).
17. Burk RW III, Guzman-Stein G, Vasconez LO. Lidocaine and epinephrine levels in tumescent technique liposuction. Plast Reconstr Surg 1996; 97(7):1379–1384.
18. Klein JA. Liposuction: anesthetic formulation of tumescent solutions. Dermatologic Clinics 1999; 17(4):751–759.
19. Klasco RK, ed. DRUGDEX(R) System. Thomson MICROMEDEX, Greenwood Village, Colorado (Edition expires 2004).
20. Schilling CG, Bank DE, Borchert BA, et al. Tetracaine, epinephrine (adrenalin), and cocaine (TAC) versus lidocaine, epinephrine, and tetracaine (LET) for anesthesia of lacerations in children. Ann Emerg Med 1995; 25(2):203–208.
21. Richards KA, Stasko T. Dermatologic surgery and the pregnant patient. Dermatol Surg 2002; 28(3):248–256.
22. Malamed SF. Handbook of Medical Emergencies in the Dental Office. 3rd ed. St. Louis: CV Mosby, 1987.
23. Steinberg MD, Block P. The use and abuse of epinephrine in local anesthetics. J Am Paediatry Assoc 1971; 61(9):341–343.
24. Gandy W. Severe epinephrine-propranolol interaction. Ann Emerg Med 1989; 18(1): 98–99.

25. Berbaum MW, Bredle DL, Futamara W. Absence of significant adverse effects from low-dose subcutaneous epinephrine in dermatologic procedures. Arch Dermatol 1997; 133(10):1318–1319.
26. Millay DJ, Larrabee WF Jr., Carpenter RL. Vasoconstrictors in facial plastic surgery. Arch Otolaryngol Head Neck Surg 1991; 117(2):160–163.
27. Smith GA, Strausbaugh SD, Harbeck-Weber C, et al. Prilocaine-phenylephrine and bupivacaine-phenylephrine topical anesthetics compared with tetracaine-adrenaline-cocaine during repair of lacerations. Am J Emerg Med 1998; 16(2):121–124.
28. Gross JB, Hartigan ML, Schaffer DW. A suitable substitute for 4% cocaine before blind nasotracheal intubation: 3% lidocaine-0.25% phenylephrine nasal spray. Anesth Analg 1984; 63(10):915–918.
29. Jones J, Greenberg L, Groudine S, et al. Clinical advisory: phenylephrine advisory panel report. Int J Pediatr Otorhinolaryngol 1998; 45(1):97–99.
30. Malhotra R, Banerjee G, Brampton W, et al. Comparison of the cardiovascular effects of 2.5% phenylephrine and 10% phenylephrine during ophthalmic surgery. Eye 1998; 12(pt 6):973–975.
31. Martindale: the complete drug reference. London: Pharmaceutical Press. Electronic Version, Thompson MICROMEDEX, Greenwood Village, Colorado, 2004 (Edition expires 2004).
32. Kishikawa K, Namiki A, Harada Y, et al. Norepinephrine prolongs tetracaine spinal anesthesia in surgical patients: a preliminary study. Anesth Analg 1993; 76(4): 772–777.
33. Kaufman E, Garfunkel A, Findler M, et al. [Emergencies evolving from local anesthesia]. Refuat Hapeh Vehashinayim 2002; 19(1):13–18, 98.
34. Dental anesthetics and the porphyric. Porphyria Educational Services Bulletin vol 1 no. 13, March 1999. Available at: http://members.tripod.com/~PorphBook/vol13 .html. Accessed August 2004.
35. Product Information: Carbocaine (R) 2% with neo-cobefrin. 2004. Cook-Waite. Manufactured for Eastman Kodak by Novocol Pharmaceuticals of Canada, Cambridge, Ontario, Canada, N1R6X3.
36. Heinonen OP, Slone D, Shapiro S. Birth Defects and Drugs in Pregnancy. Littleton, MA: Publishing Sciences Group, 1976.
37. Kam PC, Tay TM. The pharmacology of ornipressin (POR-8): a local vasoconstrictor used in surgery. Eur J Anaesthesiol 1998; 15(2):133–139.
38. Clodius L, Smahel J. POR 8, a new vasoconstrictor substitute for adrenaline in plastic surgery. Br J Plast Surg 1970; 23(1):73–76.
39. Lamont AS, Yorke P. Maximum safe dose of POR8. Anaesth Intensive Care 1987; 15(4):467.
40. Abel M, Goebel A, von Gravert H. [Supraventricular tachycardia following POR 8 (ornipressin)—administration in an infant]. Anaesthesist 1987; 36(11):653–654.
41. Kasahara M, Ichinohe T, Kaneko Y. Adenosine and amrinone reverse felypressin-induced depression of myocardial tissue oxygen tension in dogs. Can J Anaesth 2000; 47(11):1107–1113.
42. Yagiela JA. Vasoconstrictor agents for local anesthesia. Anesth Prog 1995; 42(3–4): 116–120.
43. Fitzgerald PA. Hypothalamic and pituitary hormones. In: Katzung BG, ed. Basic and Clinical Pharmacology. New York: McGraw-Hill, 2004.

44. New Zealand Medicines and Medical Devices Safety Authority. 3% Citanest® DENTAL with Octapressin®. Available at: http://www.medsafe.govt.nz/Profs/ Datasheet/c/Citanestwithoctapressininj.htm. Accessed August 2004.

45. Sunada K, Nakamura K, Yamashiro M, et al. Clinically safe dosage of felypressin for patients with essential hypertension. Anesth Prog 1996; 43(4):108–115.

46. McEvoy GK. American Society of Health-System Pharmacists. Available at: http://www.ahfsdruginformation.com

47. Chiueh CC, Kopin IJ. Centrally mediated release by cocaine of endogenous epinephrine and norepinephrine from the sympathoadrenal medullary system of unanesthetized rats. J Pharmacol Exp Ther 1978; 205(1):148–154.

48. Coleman DL, Ross TF, Naughton JL. Myocardial ischemia and infarction related to recreational cocaine use. West J Med 1982; 136(5):444–446.

49. Gay GR. Clinical management of acute and chronic cocaine poisoning. Ann Emerg Med 1982; 11(10):562–572.

50. Jatlow P. Cocaine: analysis, pharmacokinetics, and metabolic disposition. Yale J Biol Med 1988; 61(2):105–113.

51. Huang W, Vidimos A. Topical anesthetics in dermatology. J Am Acad Dermatol 2000; 43(2 pt 1):286–298.

52. Barash PG, Kopriva CJ, Langou R, et al. Is cocaine a sympathetic stimulant during general anesthesia? JAMA 1980; 243(14):1437–1439.

53. Terndrup TE, Walls HC, Mariani PJ, et al. Plasma cocaine and tetracaine levels following application of topical anesthesia in children. Ann Emerg Med 1992; 21(2):162–166.

54. Bonadio WA, Wagner VR. Adrenaline-cocaine gel topical anesthetic for dermal laceration repair in children. Ann Emerg Med 1992; 21(12):1435–1438.

55. Nakamura GR, Noguchi TT. Fatalities from cocaine overdoses in Los Angeles County. Clin Toxicol 1981; 18(8):895–905.

56. Schubert CJ, Wason S. Cocaine toxicity in an infant following intranasal instillation of a four percent cocaine solution. Pediatr Emerg Care 1992; 8(2):82–83.

57. Brogan WC III, Lange RA, Kim AS, et al. Alleviation of cocaine-induced coronary vasoconstriction by nitroglycerin. J Am Coll Cardiol 1991; 18(2):581–586.

58. Daya MR, Burton BT, Schleiss MR, et al. Recurrent seizures following mucosal application of TAC. Ann Emerg Med 1988; 17(6):646–648.

59. Young SL, Vosper HJ, Phillips SA. Cocaine: its effects on maternal and child health. Pharmacotherapy 1992; 12(1):2–17.

60. Slutsker L. Risks associated with cocaine use during pregnancy. Obstet Gynecol 1992; 79(5 pt 1):778–789.

61. Graham K, Feigenbaum A, Pastuszak A, et al. Pregnancy outcome and infant development following gestational cocaine use by social cocaine users in Toronto, Canada. Clin Invest Med 1992; 15(4):384–394.

62. Hearn WL, Rose S, Wagner J, et al. Cocaethylene is more potent than cocaine in mediating lethality. Pharmacol Biochem Behav 1991; 39(2):531–533.

63. Cederholm I, Akerman B, Evers H. Local analgesic and vascular effects of intradermal ropivacaine and bupivacaine in various concentrations with and without addition of adrenaline in man. Acta Anaesthesiol Scand 1994; 38(4):322–327.

64. Kopacz DJ, Carpenter RL, Mackey DC. Effect of ropivacaine on cutaneous capillary blood flow in pigs. Anesthesiology 1989; 71(1):69–74.

65. Product Information: Regetine, phentolamine. 1998. East Hanover, NJ, Novartis Pharmaceuticals.

66. Goldstein I, Carson C, Rosen R, et al. Vasomax for the treatment of male erectile dysfunction. World J Urol 2001; 19(1):51–56.

67. Hinterberger JW, Kintzi HE. Phentolamine reversal of epinephrine-induced digital vasospasm. How to save an ischemic finger. Arch Fam Med 1994; 3(2):193–195.

68. Wu G, Calamel PM, Shedd DP. The hazards of injecting local anesthetic solutions with epinephrine into flaps: experimental study. Plast Reconstr Surg 1978; 62(3): 396–403.

69. Wolfort S, Rohrich RJ, Handren J, et al. The effect of epinephrine in local anesthesia on the survival of full- and split-thickness skin grafts: an experimental study. Plast Reconstr Surg 1990; 86(3):535–540.

70. Fazio MJ, Zitelli JA. Full-thickness skin grafts. Clinical observations on the impact of using epinephrine in local anesthesia of the donor site. Arch Dermatol 1995; 131(6): 691–694.

71. Atabey A, Galdino G, El Shahat A, et al. The effects of tumescent solutions containing lidocaine and epinephrine on skin flap survival in rats. Ann Plast Surg 2004; 53(1):70–72.

72. Irwin C. In: Lundberg A, Moody P. www.nursing.uiowa.edu/sites/PedsPain/Procedur/Tacnurse.htm. Accessed August 2004.

73. Vinci RJ, Fish SS. Efficacy of topical anesthesia in children. Arch Pediatr Adolesc Med 1996; 150(5):466–469.

74. Smith GA, Strausbaugh SD, Harbeck-Weber C, et al. New non-cocaine-containing topical anesthetics compared with tetracaine-adrenaline-cocaine during repair of lacerations. Pediatrics 1997; 100(5):825–830.

75. Ernst AA, Marvez-Valls E, Nick TG, et al. LAT (lidocaine-adrenaline-tetracaine) versus TAC (tetracaine-adrenaline-cocaine) for topical anesthesia in face and scalp lacerations. Am J Emerg Med 1995; 13(2):151–154.

76. Altinyazar HC, Ozdemir H, Koca R, et al. Epinephrine in digital block: color Doppler flow imaging. Dermatol Surg 2004; 30(4 pt 1):508–511.

77. Keel D, Goldman MP. Tumescent anesthesia in ambulatory phlebectomy: addition of epinephrine. Dermatol Surg 1999; 25(5):371–372.

78. Ramirez OM, Galdino G. Does tumescent infiltration have a deleterious effect on undermined skin flaps? Plast Reconstr Surg 1999; 104(7):2269–2272.

79. Breuninger H, Hobbach PS, Schimek F. Ropivacaine: an important anesthetic agent for slow infusion and other forms of tumescent anesthesia. Dermatol Surg 1999; 25(10): 799–802.

80. Moehrle M, Breuninger H. Dermatosurgery using subcutaneous infusion anesthesia with prilocaine and ropivacaine in children. Pediatr Dermatol 2001; 18(6):469–472.

81. Moses S. Family Practice Notebook, LLC, http://www.fpnotebook.com/NEU192.htm. Accessed August 2004, Revised 09/08/2007.

82. Hoffman BB. Adrenoceptor-activating and other sympathomimetic drugs. In: Katzung BG, ed. New York: McGraw-Hill, 2004.

3

Topical Anesthetics

S. 't Kint

*Department of Dermatology, University Hospital
Brussels (UZ Brussel), Brussels, Belgium*

D. Roseeuw

*Department of Dermatology, University Hospital
Brussels (UZ Brussel), Brussels, Belgium*

INTRODUCTION

Topical anesthetics have become more and more important in dermatologic surgery. Their importance has grown with the recent evolution in laser surgery and surgical procedures. They provide a safe, effective, and painless cutaneous analgesia with slow onset but prolonged duration (1,2).

Pharmacology of the anesthetics consists of ester- or amide-derived agents (3). The ester anesthetics have an ester linkage between the aromatic ring and the intermediate chain. They are hydrolyzed by plasma cholinesterase forming para-amino benzoic acid (PABA), which is a potent allergen. Ester anesthetics are contraindicated in patients with known allergies to PABA, hair dyes, and sulphonamides.

The amide anesthetics have an amide linkage between the aromatic ring and the intermediate chain. They are primarily enzymatically metabolized in the liver. Amide anesthetics are rare sensitizers (Fig. 1).

The target for cutaneous analgesia is the dermis since it contains free nerve endings and blood vessels. Topical anesthetic inhibits the sodium influx of

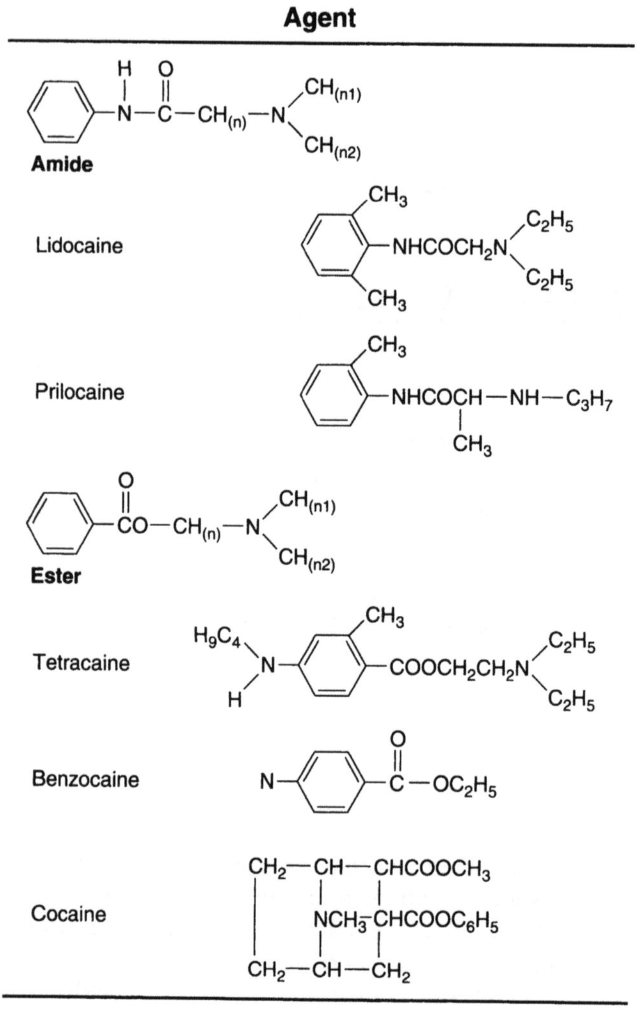

Agent

Figure 1 Structures of topical anesthetics.

sodium channels of the nerve synaps, thereby increasing the threshold for nerve excitation until the inability to produce an action potential. This mechanism blocks the nerve endings and leads to the prevention of the initiation and transmission of nerve impulse (4).

The potency of the product is determined by the lipid solubility of the anesthetic, the protein-binding capacity, the acid ionization constant, and the vasodilatory profile (5).

TOPICAL ANESTHETICS

EMLA (Eutectic Mixture of Local Anesthetics)

EMLA is a eutectic mixture of the local anesthetics lidocaine 2.5% and prilocaine 2.5% (6). The term "eutectic" refers to the fact that the mixture has a melting point lower than that of either anesthetic alone (7). Thus it consists as an emulsion with a dispersed phase (the mixture) and a continuous phase (water). The absorption is therefore enhanced by the water component.

Formula: Lidocaine 25 mg
Prilocaine 25 mg
Polyoxyethylene ester (emulsifier) 19 mg
Carboxypolymethylene (thickener) 10 mg
Sodium hydroxide to pH 9
Purified H_2O to 1 g

EMLA must be applied under an occlusive dressing to facilitate the absorption in the skin. A minimal application time of one hour is recommended for minor procedures, except for more painful procedures where the duration must be minimally two hours (8).

The penetration depth is 3 mm after one hour and 5 mm after two hours application time (9). The duration of the cutaneous analgesia after application is 180 minutes. Local blood flow and epidermal and dermal thickness are important factors concerning the efficacy of the agent (10).

EMLA is ineffective on palmar and plantar surfaces due to the thickened stratum corneum. On mucosal surfaces, the application approaches levels similar to parenteral administration. A shorter application time of 15 minutes provides an efficient analgesia on mucosal surfaces.

The recommended dose is based upon the patient's age, body weight, and application area. Guidelines recommend that in children weighing less than 10 kg, and older than 12 months including neonates, application should be limited to 2 g and applied to an area smaller than 100 cm^2. In children weighing 10 to 20 kg the maximum dose is 10 g and should be limited to an area of 100 cm^2 (11,12).

Eutectic lidocaine/prilocaine has been used in multiple indications. It is effective in relieving the pain prior to arterial cannulation, venipuncture, punch biopsies, split-skin graft harvesting, curettage of molluscum contagiosum, laser treatment of facial port-wine stains with the pulsed dye laser, Q switched Nd: YAG laser, surgical debridement of leg ulcers, removal of condylomata accuminata, epilation and chemical peels. It is useful as adjunct to local anesthetics in dermabrasion and laser resurfacing (13–15).

The greatest risk in the use of EMLA is methemoglobinemia, attributed to metabolites of prilocaine (4-hydroxy-2-methylalaniline and *o*-toluidine)

(16). Use of EMLA is contraindicated in infants less than three months of age because of low levels of erythrocyte methemoglobin reductase, in congenital or idiopathic methemoglobinemia, concomitant use of methemoglobinemia-inducing agents (sulphonamide derivates, phenytoin, phenobarbital, dapsone, benzocaine, and acetaminophen agents) and in patients with glucose-6-phoshate deficiency.

Minor side effects are mild and transient, and resolve spontaneously. They are limited to the application site: erythema (30%), paleness (37%), changed ability to feel hot or cold, edema (7%), itching (2%), and rash (1%).

Hypersensitivity reactions and systemic toxicity are very rare. However, some cases have been reported to the prilocaine component of the mixture.

ELA-Max

ELA-Max is a prilocaine-free topical anesthetic containing 4% lidocaine encapsulated in a liposomal vehicle (17). The lipid carrier system benefits the delivery of lidocaine into the dermis, providing sustained release (18,19).

> Formula: Lidocaine 40 mg
> Vitamine E acetate
> Propylene glycol
> Benzyl alcohol
> Cholesterol
> Carbomer 940
> Triethanolamine
> Polysorbate 80
> Purified H_2O

The application time recommended is 60 minutes, with an increased anesthetic effect 30 minutes after removal. There is no consensus regarding the use of ELA-Max under occlusion. Clinical studies comparing EMLA and ELA-Max showed both to be equally effective. However, ELA-Max has a faster onset and a longer duration (20). The liposomal delivery system enhances the penetration of encapsulated drug into the dermis and protecting it from metabolic degradation.

In children weighing less than 20 kg, a single application should be limited to an area less than 100 cm^2 (12). Due to the greater absorption, ELA-Max should not be applied to mucous membranes. There have been no studies to evaluate the risk of application and toxic effect on membranes.

The anesthetic efficacity has been studied in venipuncture, laser surgery, and in TCA peels (21,22). It relieves pain after superficial burns, irritation of the skin, and skin abrasions.

Till now there is little evidence of major side effects. Due to the absence of prilocaine, the risk of methemoglobinemia is minimalized.

Minor side effects on the application side are transient erythema and paleness.

Further studies are recommended to evaluate the efficacy and safety of this topical agent.

Amethocaine

Amethocaine contains 4% tetracaine gel. Tetracaine is a lipophilic molecule, which crosses the stratum corneum more rapidly to affect the nerve endings, and who allows the agent to form a depot in the stratum corneum (23). This explains the rapid onset and the long duration of action (24,25).

Amethocaine must be applied under occlusion. The minimal application time is 40 minutes, and the duration of cutaneous analgesia after removal is four hours (26).

The recommended adult dose is 50 mg. The use on mucous membranes has not been studied and should be used with great caution.

Amethocaine has proven its efficacy for venous cannulation and pulsed dye treatment for port-wine stains (27–30).

Adverse events reported include local erythema, pruritus, and edema. Amethocaine is an ester-derived anesthetic and undergoes hydrolysis into PABA, which is a potent allergen.

Topicaine

Topicaine is a 4% lidocaine solution in a gel microemulsion delivering a rapid anesthesia with a prolonged duration (31). It must be applied under an occlusive dressing 30 to 60 minutes prior to treatment (32,33).

Topicaine has been used as a topical anesthetic prior to electrolysis, laser hair removal, and in laser-induced pain stimuli.

The maximum area of application should not exceed 600 cm^2 in adults and 100 cm^2 in children.

There are only reports of minor side effects such as erythema, blanching, and edema. No systemic toxicity or hypersensitivity reactions are known.

S-Caine Patch

S-caine patch contains a 1/1 eutectic mixture of lidocaine (2.5%) and tetracaine (2.5%) with an oxygen-activated heat element, which enhances the penetration into the dermis (13,34,35).

The patch must not be used under occlusion and an application time of 30 minutes is required to obtain adequate anesthesia (13,14,36).

Promising results are viewed for shave biopsies and venipuncture.

CONCLUSION

Topical anesthetics are a new advance for pain relief prior to dermatological procedures.

It decreases the anxiety of the patients, especially the children, since there is no longer the need for anesthetic injections. Therefore a greater compliance is obtained during the preparation and the onset of the surgical act.

EMLA is worldwide the most used topical anesthetic that enhances our experience. It is a safe, effective, low-cost product with long-duration effect. The disadvantage is the slow onset of action and the possibility to induce methemoglobinemia in neonates.

This has led to the development of new topical anesthetics, where the renewal remains the specialized drug delivery systems that give a faster onset of action, longer duration, and selectivity to the dermis without systemic toxicity.

However more data are required to evaluate the safety and the efficacy of these agents.

REFERENCES

1. Keyes PD, Tallon JM, Rizos J. Topical anesthesia. Can Fam Physician 1998; 44: 2152–2156.
2. Kundu S, Achar S. Principles of office anesthesia: part II. Topical anesthesia. Am Fam Physician 2002; 66:99–102.
3. Covino BG. Pharmacology of local anaesthetic agents. Br J Anaesth 1986; 58: 701–716.
4. Friedman PM, Fogelman JP, Nouri K. Comparative study of the efficacy of four topical anesthetics. Dermatol Surg 1999; 25:950–954.
5. Schaefer H, Zesch A, Stuttgen G. Skin Permeability. Heidelberg: Springer-Verlag, 1982:604–607.
6. Lycka BA. EMLA: a new and effective topical anesthetic. J Dermatol Surg Oncol 1992; 18:859–862.
7. Buckley MM, Benfield P. Eutectic lidocaine/prilocaine cream. Drugs 1993; 46:126–151.
8. Lycka B. Medical indications for using a topical anesthetic. Perspect Pain Management 1991; 1:9–12.
9. Sarifakioglu N, Terzioglu A, Cigsar B. EMLA and ear surgery: is it possible to achieve full-thickness anesthesia with EMLA? Dermatol Surg 2004; 30:395–398.
10. Bjerring P, Andersen PH, Arendt-Nielsen L. Vascular response of human skin after analgesia with EMLA cream. Br J Anaesth 1989; 63:655–560.
11. Lillieborg S, Otterbom I, Ahlen K. Topical anesthesia in neonates, infants and children. Br J Anaesth 2004; 92:450–451.
12. Chen BK, Eichenfield LF. Pediatric anesthesia in dermatologic surgery: when hand-holding is not enough. Dermatol Surg 2001; 27:101–118.
13. Doshi SN, Friedman PM, Marquez DK. Thirty-minute application of the S-caine peel prior to nonablative laser treatment. Dermatol Surg 2003; 29:1008–1011.
14. Chen JZ, Alexiades-Armenakas MR, Bernstein LJ, et al. Two randomize, double-blind, placebo-controlled studies evaluating the S-caine peel for induction of local

anesthesia before long-pulsed Nd:YAG laser therapy for leg veins. Dermatol Surg 2003; 29(10):1012–1018.

15. Vesterager L, Petersen KP, Nielsen R. EMLA-induced analgesia inferior to lignocaine infiltration in curettage of common warts—a randomized study. Dermatology 1994; 188:32–35.

16. Vessely MB, Zitsch RP III. Topical anesthetic-induced methemoglobinemia: a case report and review of the literature. Otolaryngol Head Neck Surg 1993; 108:763–767.

17. Tang MB, Goon AT, Goh CL. Study on the efficacy of ELA-Max (4% liposomal lidocaine) compared with EMLA cream (eutectic mixture of local anesthetics) using thermosensory threshold analysis in adult volunteers. J Dermatolog Treat 2004; 15(2): 84–87.

18. Koppel RA, Coleman KM, Coleman WP. The efficacy of EMLA versus ELA-Max for pain relief in medium depth chemical peeling: a clinical and histopathologic evaluation. Dermatol Surg 2000; 26:61–64.

19. Schmid MH, Korting HC. Liposomes: a drug carrier system for topical treatment in dermatology. Crit Rev Ther Drug Carrier Syst 1994; 11:97–118.

20. Friedman PM, Mafong EA, Friedman ES. Topical anesthetics Update: EMLA and Beyond. Dermatol Surg 2001; 27:1019–1026.

21. Eremia S, Newman N. Topical anesthesia for laser hair removal: comparison of spot size and 755 nm versus 800 nm wavelengths. Dermatol Surg 2000; 26:667–669.

22. Altman DA. Gildenberg SR. High-energy pulsed light source hair removal device used to evaluate the onset of action of a new topical anesthetic. Dermatol Surg 1999; 25:816–818.

23. Fisher R, Hung O, Mezei M. Topical anaesthesia of intact skin: liposome-encapsulated tetraca vs EMLA. Br J Anaesth 1998; 81(6):972–973.

24. Holmes MV, Dawe RS, Ferguson J. A randomized, double-blind, placebo-controlled study of the efficacy of tetracaine gel (Ametop) for pain relief during topical photodynamic therapy. Br J Dermatol 2004; 150:337–340.

25. Arevalo MI, Escribano E, Calpena A. Rapid skin anesthesia using a new topical amethocaine formulation: a preclinical study. Anesth Analg 2004; 98(5):1407–1412.

26. Jain A, Rutter N, Ratnayaka M. Topical amethocaine gel for pain relief of heel prick blood sampling: a randomized double-blind controlled trial. Arch Dis Child Fetal Neonatal Ed 2001; 84(1):F56–F59.

27. Aaron SD, Vandenheem KL, Naftel SA. Topical tetracaine prior to arterial puncture: a randomized, placebo-controlled clinical trial. Respir Med 2003; 97(11):1195–1199.

28. Long CP, McCafferty DF, Sittlington NM. Randomized trial of novel tetracaine patch to provide local anaesthesia in neonates undergoing venepuncture. Br J Anaesth 2003; 91(4):514–521.

29. Moore J. No more tears: a randomized controlled double-blind trial of Amethocaine gel vs. placebo in the management of procedural pain in neonates. J Adv Nurs 2001; 34(4):475–482.

30. Jain A, Rutter N. Topical amethocaine gel in the newborn infant: how soon does it work and how long does it last? Arch Dis Child Fetal Neonatal Ed 2000; 83(3):F211–F214.

31. Goldmann RD. ELA-Max: a new topical lidocaine formulation. Ann Pharmacother 2004; 38:892–894.

32. Zempsky WT, Parkinson TM. Lidocaine iontophoresis for topical anesthesia before dermatologic procedures in children: a randomize controlled trial. Pediatr Dermatol 2003; 20:364–368.
33. Zempsky WT, Parkinson TM. Lidocaine iontophoresis for local anesthesia before shave biopsy. Dermatol Surg 2003; 29:627–630.
34. Meier T, Faust M, Huppe M. Reduction of chronic pain for non-postherpetic peripheral neuropathies after topical treatment with a lidocaine patch. Schmerz 2004; 18:172–178.
35. Long CP, McCafferty DF, Sittlington NM. Randomized trial of novel tetracaine patch to provide local anaesthesia in neonates undergoing venepuncture. Br J Anaesth 2003; 91:514–518.
36. Davies PS, Galer BS. Review of lidocaine patch 5% studies in the treatment of postherpetic neuralgia. Drugs 2004; 64:937–947.

4

Local Infiltration Anesthesia

Christie T. Ammirati

*Department of Dermatology, Penn State Milton
S. Hershey Medical Center, Hershey,
Pennsylvania, U.S.A.*

George J. Hruza

*Laser and Dermatologic Surgery Center, Town
and Country and Department of Dermatology
and Otolaryngology/Head and Neck Surgery,
St. Louis University School of Medicine,
St. Louis, Missouri, U.S.A.*

Having occasion, however, about the end of 1853, to endeavor to remove a nævus by injection with the acid solution of perchloride of iron, I procured one of the elegant little syringes constructed for this purpose by Mr. Ferguson of Giltspur Street, London. While using this instrument for the nævus, it occurred to me that it might supply the means of bringing some narcotic to bear more directly than I had hitherto been able to accomplish on the affected nerve in neuralgia. I resolved to make the attempt and did not long lack the opportunity.

Alexander Wood, 1855 (1)

HISTORY

Before infiltrative anesthesia could be performed effectively, an appropriate delivery device had to be invented and an effective local anesthetic had to be isolated. Interestingly, it was the ancient Javanese practice of using darts to deliver poison that provided the first experimental model for subcutaneous infiltration. In 1809, François Magendie studied the systemic effects of this poison (later shown to be strychnine) after "spearing" it into the buttocks of dogs on the tip of a wooden barb (2). Despite initial interest in his findings, the concept of subcutaneous delivery was abandoned for nearly a quarter of a century. In 1836, the French physician G.V. Lafargue attempted to treat his trigeminal neuralgia by performing multiple punctures along the course of the affected nerve with a lancet dipped in morphine solution (3). He reported transient cure of his pain and, despite noting a "strong desire to sleep," mistakenly attributed his success to the local and not systemic effects of the morphine. Multiple versions of the hypodermic syringe were introduced over the next 20 years, and the modern-day version cannot be clearly attributed to one person. However, we do know that the first person to report what was believed to be local analgesia from subcutaneous infiltration of a substance with a hypodermic syringe was Alexander Wood in 1855 (1). Similar to his predecessors, he mistook the systemic opiate effects of morphine as local and was only hindered by the lack of an effective anesthetic.

> Hardly recognized as an internal remedy, and described as a poison of such great power, it was with no small anxiety that, in 1859, I first injected atropine beneath the skin.
>
> Charles Hunter, 1863 (4)

As the development of the hypodermic syringe progressed, so did the understanding of the effects produced by infiltration of various medications. The majority of studies at that time focused on morphine and other opiate preparations, but despite their well-known toxicities, subcutaneous atropine and strychnine were also popular treatments for neuralgia. In truth, none of these medications induced local anesthesia, and any effect they had was central (2). It is ironic that one of the first injectable agents that actually decreased local sensation was not recognized as such for many years. In 1875, Lafitte injected what he thought was morphine into a painful neuroma with immediate relief (5). He later discovered that his servant had stolen the morphine and replaced it with water. He performed further studies and confirmed his findings, but his peers discounted any anesthetic effect from the infiltration of water as purely psychological.

Around the same time Wood published his hypodermic method for treating neuralgia, the Austrian naturalist Karl von Scherzer passed through Peru on a worldwide expedition. He noted the practice of chewing coca leaves that was pervasive among the indigenous people and sent a sample to the German chemist Albert Niemann. In 1860, Niemann purified the active component and named it cocaine (6). While the term "cocaine" was new, archaeological studies in Ecuador indicate that human ingestion of the coca leaf can be traced back for at least 5000 years (7). There is evidence to suggest that ancient Incan healers were aware of the anesthetic effects from chewing coca leaves, but the first known written reference was in 1653 by the Spanish Jesuit Bernabé Cobo.

And this happen'd to me once, that I repaired to a barber to have a tooth pull'd, that had work'd loose and ached, and the barber told me he would be sorry to pull it because it was sound and healthy; and a monk friend of mine who happen'd to be there and overhearing, advised me to chew for a few days on Coca. As I did, indeed, soon to find my toothache gone.

Bernabé Cobo, 1653 (8)

Interest in cocaine's local effects would not resurface for almost 200 years. Although Niemann's 1860 report mentioned that in addition to a bitter taste, brief contact with the extract numbed his tongue, it was not until 1884 that Carl Koller performed the first surgery under cocaine local anesthesia (9). Koller was a friend and contemporary of Sigmund Freud, who at that time was studying cocaine's stimulant effect and its potential as a cure for morphine addiction. During one of these studies, they noted how numb the tongue and mucosa became after contact with cocaine. This led Koller to begin experimenting with cocaine solution as a topical anesthetic for the eye. After confirming its effect on animals and later his own eyes, he performed the first operation for glaucoma with cocaine local anesthesia in September 1884 (10).

Recall that up to this time, subcutaneous injection had only been considered as a treatment for existing pain and not to preempt it. After reading of Koller's success on mucous membranes, the American surgeon William Halsted began to experiment with cocaine injection around peripheral nerve roots on himself and his coworkers (11). Within a month, he reported the first alveolar nerve block that was sufficient to allow for painless tooth extraction. Next he removed a congenital forehead lesion after performing a supraorbital nerve block. He then progressed to brachial plexus and posterior tibial blocks and was able to demonstrate conclusively that proximal injection of a nerve could impede distal pain impulses from an extremity (12). Within a year, Halsted had performed more than a thousand operations after injecting cocaine and became the recognized founder of regional anesthesia. Unfortunately, his self-experimentation had also left him and his coworkers with lifelong drug addictions.

Infiltration anesthesia differs from topical anesthesia in that the anesthetic is not applied to the surface and allowed to diffuse; rather it is injected directly into or around the wound. It differs from regional anesthesia by striving to block cutaneous nerves within the surgical field and not targeting individual nerves to provide distal loss of sensation. From a collection of his unpublished papers, it appears that William Halsted may have been the first to perform infiltrative surgical anesthesia. He described removing nevi and draining abscesses after infiltration of cocaine or distilled water directly into lesions as early as 1886, but was of "ill health" or, as others have suggested, too impaired by his addiction to cocaine to report his findings (13).

To Schleich very properly goes the credit he has received in as much as my work, owing to ill health, was not published.

William Halsted, 1920 (13)

The honor of formally introducing the concept of infiltrative surgical anesthesia goes to Carl Ludwig Schleich (1859–1922), who presented his method at the 1892 Annual Congress of the German Surgical Society (14). In contrast to Halsted's popular nerve block technique, Schleich did not target individual nerves to create distal anesthesia. Instead, he placed overlapping injections of cocaine directly into the surgical field to block local nerve endings. He added additional comfort by using topical ether to cool the skin before injection. He was familiar with the potential toxicity of cocaine, and for safety he recommended starting with dilute cocaine and reserving concentrated solutions for inflamed tissues. Although this was a monumental discovery, which would have a profound impact on the practice of surgery, Schleich was a controversial physician with strong opinions. Schleich's presentation of his technique to members of the German Surgical Society was filled with accusations and inflammatory statements, which only served to incite his audience. As with so many medical discoveries that are tainted by the personality of their innovator, Schleich's method was not met with initial approval and in fact he was forced to leave the podium before finishing his presentation (15). After a colorful career, he died in 1922 in a Berlin sanatorium, a reputed victim of alcohol and morphine addiction.

> Confused between hate and affection, his character swings in history.
>
> August Bier, 1922, regarding his colleague
> Carl Ludwig Schleich (16)

DEFINITION

Infiltrative anesthesia is the intradermal or subcutaneous infiltration of an anesthetic either directly into the surgical site (direct infiltration) or circumferentially around the surgical field (field block). Infiltration of an anesthetic directly below a lesion creates a small ring of anesthesia around its base that is sufficient to obtain a shave or punch biopsy. Another form of local infiltration is the field block where anesthesia is injected parallel to the surgical margins but not directly into the lesion. This method is particularly useful for infected wounds to reduce the spread of contamination or subcutaneous lesions that may be hidden by tumescence. It also reduces the chance of injecting directly into a cyst and causing rupture. The field block technique can be extrapolated to the ear, nose, and scalp, where circumferential infiltration around the base anesthetizes nearly the entire extremity.

Arguably, the most important aspects of infiltrative anesthesia are deciding whether it will provide sufficient anesthesia for the proposed surgery and which agent should be used. Absolute contraindications such as previous hypersensitivity reactions are self-evident. However, it requires critical assessment and experience to determine if the anesthetic requirements of a large lesion will exceed the maximum allowable dosage. For example, an 80-year-old cachectic woman, weighing 100 lb, presents for excision of a cumbersome and painful 15-cm lipoma on her back. She has unstable angina, chronic obstructive pulmonary disease, and uncontrolled severe hypertension that preclude the use of general anesthesia or local anesthesia containing epinephrine. The back is not amenable to regional nerve block and given her weight, the safe volume of subcutaneous 1% plain lidocaine (4.5 mg/kg) must be kept below 20 mL. An excellent solution would be to use 0.5% lidocaine, which would double the allowable volume, or even tumescent anesthesia. However, these options must be considered before surgery is begun and not midway through the procedure after maximum levels have been achieved.

REDUCING PAIN

Once it has been decided that the proposed surgery can be performed safely under local anesthesia, there are several simple measures that can make the procedure less painful (Table 1). In general, pain from local anesthesia can be divided into pain from the needle stick and pain due to infiltration, either by distention of the tissue or from contact with the anesthetic itself. Pain from the

Table 1 Methods to Decrease Pain of Infiltrative Anesthesia

Decrease pain from needle stick

- Ice
- Cryogen cooling
- Topical anesthetic
- Small gauge needle (28 or 30 gauge)
- Inject into a pore or follicle
- "One-stick" method

Decrease pain from infiltration

- Small-volume syringe
- Deep dermal injection
- Slow infiltration
- Warm, neutralized anesthetic
- Mechanical stimulation (pinching, rubbing)
- Inject bacteriostatic saline first

Psychological support

- Verbal distraction
- Handholding
- Music
- Calm atmosphere
- Keeping the needle out of sight
- Anxiolytics when necessary

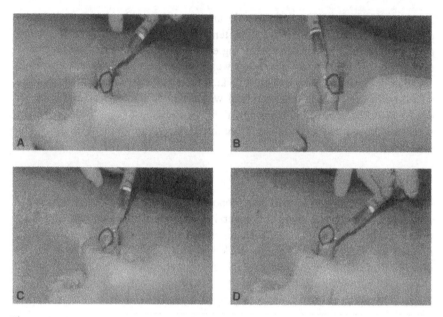

Figure 1 One-stick method: After initial infiltration, the ring of anesthesia is advanced systematically by inserting the needle into skin that is already anesthetized. This is continued in a stepwise fashion until the entire field is encircled. The skin is pinched simultaneously to provide distracting stimulus. Note the proper placement of the surgeon's fingers during this maneuver to prevent accidental injury.

needle stick can be limited by using the smallest gauge needle possible and anesthetizing the surface of the skin with ice, refrigerant sprays, cold air, or topical anesthetic creams. Distracting stimuli such as pinching or vibrating the skin can also be helpful. Ideally, the patient should feel only one needle stick, despite the size of the area that requires anesthesia. This "one-stick method" is achieved by injecting anesthesia systematically through previously anesthetized skin (Fig. 1). A 1-inch needle can help reduce the number of needle sticks when anesthetizing large lesions. If multiple lesions are to be anesthetized, the needle can become dull with repetitive passage through the skin and should be changed if resistance is noted.

Modifying the depth and speed of infiltration can reduce pain from the distention of tissue. Rapid injection into the superficial dermis and creating "peau d'orange" elicits immediate anesthesia but distends the tissue causing unnecessary pain (17). This is particularly true for areas with limited room for expansion such as the scalp, nose, palms, and soles (18). Slow injection into the deep dermis or fat is far less painful, but it may take a few minutes before the overlying superficial tissues are anesthetized. A thin 30-g needle and small-volume 1- to 5-mL syringe can help maintain a slow, steady speed of injection.

The anesthetic solution itself can cause pain upon contact with the tissue, regardless of the speed and depth in which it is infiltrated. Warming it to body temperature and neutralizing the pH can reduce the pain significantly (19). Nerve endings are exquisitely sensitive to cold and, along with decreasing the pain and increasing the speed of onset, warming lidocaine to body temperature prolongs the duration of anesthesia (20). Lidocaine has a tendency to precipitate out of solution. As such, commercial preparations of plain lidocaine are mildly acidic (6.5 pH) to prolong their shelf life. Lidocaine with epinephrine requires further acidification (pH 3.5–5.0) to retard the oxidation of epinephrine. This acidity makes infiltration of lidocaine with epinephrine more painful than plain lidocaine and much more painful than normal saline (21). Buffering lidocaine with epinephrine by adding sodium bicarbonate in a 1:10 ratio neutralizes the pH and markedly decreases pain (Table 2). The combination of warming and buffering has a synergistic effect, reducing pain beyond that of either modification alone (22). However, neutralizing the pH and warming the solution decreases the stability of epinephrine (23). To assure sufficient residual epinephrine activity for effective vasoconstriction, buffered lidocaine with epinephrine should be used within 24 hours if kept at room temperature or within 1 week if refrigerated (23,24).

Another aspect of pain during infiltration lies within the anesthetic itself and is independent of pH or additives. For example, infiltration of lidocaine is far less

Table 2 Modified Anesthetic Solutions

Buffered lidocaine 1:10 (29)

- 5 mL of 8.4% sodium bicarbonate in 45 mL of lidocaine. Refrigerate or discard after 24 h if kept at room temperature

Dilute lidocaine in bacteriostatic saline 1:10 (29)

- 3 mL lidocaine in 27 mL bacteriostatic saline

Bacteriostatic saline with epinephrine 1:100,000 (29)

- 0.3 mL of 1:1000 epinephrine in 30 mL of bacteriostatic saline

Hyaluronidase in lidocaine 5 IU/mL (42)

- 150 IU of hyaluronidase in 30 mL of 1% lidocaine

Dilute diphenhydramine (45)

- 1% diphenhydramine: 1 mL of 50 mg/mL (5% solution) in 4 mL of sterile saline
- 0.5% diphenhydramine: 1 mL of 50 mg/mL (5% solution) in 9 mL of sterile saline

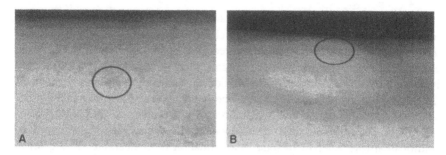

Figure 2   Dermatofibroma on the lower extremity (**A**) before and (**B**) after infiltration of bacteriostatic saline, creating the tense dermal wheal necessary for effective anesthesia with this agent.

painful than bupivacaine or diphenhydramine (25). One percent diphenhydramine provides an alternative to patients with hypersensitivity to amide-linked anesthetics but is very painful to inject and takes approximately 20 minutes to be effective (26). It is also complicated by delayed sedation, and concentrations >1% may cause cutaneous necrosis (Table 2) (27). An interesting alternative to amides or diphenyl compounds that provides nearly painless infiltration is bacteriostatic saline, which is a solution of 0.9% sodium chloride with 0.9% benzyl alcohol. The anesthetic properties of benzyl alcohol, which is an opium alkaloid, have been known since 1918 (28). Bacteriostatic saline can provide 2 to 5 minutes of anesthesia, which is sufficient for very superficial procedures such as shave biopsy, scissor excision, or curettage. Epinephrine can be added to lengthen the duration but does not create adequate anesthesia to allow for more invasive procedures such as deep punch biopsies or surgical excisions (Table 2). The method of delivery for bacteriostatic saline is different from that of other local anesthetics (21). To be effective, bacteriostatic saline must be given in a volume large enough to create a tense dermal wheal; typically this volume is two to three times what would ordinarily be used for lidocaine (Fig. 2).

An excellent means of decreasing pain is to use agents with complimentary attributes in combination or tandem. Lidocaine diluted 1:10 with bacteriostatic saline is markedly less painful than lidocaine alone and provides approximately 20 minutes of anesthesia (29). Bacteriostatic saline also serves as an excellent diluent for corticosteroids and botulinum toxin, where it can significantly decrease the pain of infiltration. For areas that require epinephrine vasoconstriction, plain lidocaine can be injected before lidocaine with epinephrine. Anesthetizing first with lidocaine can also abolish the pain from injecting long-acting bupivacaine.

The combination of ice, bacteriostatic saline, lidocaine, and bupivacaine can provide nearly painless, immediate, and prolonged anesthesia (30). In this method, the skin is first chilled with an ice pack or other cryogen for several minutes. Once chilled, the skin is injected immediately with sufficient volumes of bacteriostatic saline to cause tissue blanching and tumescence (31). This is followed by infiltration of buffered lidocaine with epinephrine. For more complex and lengthy procedures, such as Mohs micrographic surgery, infiltration of lidocaine is followed by bupivacaine.

Heightened anxiety and distress are known to lower a patient's threshold for painful stimuli (32). The first step to identifying overly anxious patients is to create a setting that is conducive to their disclosure of any apprehensions that they may have. The best time to lay the groundwork for this relationship is during the preoperative consult, where these concerns can be addressed. Patients with a history of previous anxiety attacks or syncopal episodes associated with needles may benefit from a preoperative anxiolytic.

The atmosphere in the surgical suite should be calm and soothing. The room should be organized to avoid last-minute running around for instruments and kept at a comfortable temperature. Personnel should be unhurried, courteous, and professional. Patients should be given the option to listen to music that they select, and extraneous noises such as inappropriately loud conversation, alarms, and intercoms should be kept to a minimum (33). Once the patient is positioned comfortably, the surgeon should provide verbal reassurance and keep the needle from sight. All injections should be done with the patient recumbent to minimize the potential of a vasovagal reaction. It may also be helpful to have an assistant hold or massage the patient's hand during infiltration of the anesthetic (34–36). Distracting physical stimuli, such as stretching, rubbing, vibrating, or pinching the surrounding skin during infiltration, can significantly decrease the pain from infiltration of anesthesia (37). This manipulation stimulates local sensory nerves and partially blocks the transmission of painful impulses (32). Care must be taken that the surgeon's fingers are kept safe from accidental needle stick while performing these maneuvers (Fig. 1).

FACTORS AFFECTING QUALITY OF INFILTRATIVE ANESTHESIA

pH

Local anesthetic solutions exist in water-soluble ionized (cation) and lipid-soluble non-ionized (base) form. The relative proportion of these two forms is governed by the dissociation constant (pKa) of the anesthetic and the pH of its environment. The pKa is defined as the pH where the ratio of ionized to nonionized form is equal. The nonionized form is lipid soluble and able to diffuse into the nerve fiber. Most local anesthetics are weak bases with a pKa in the range of 7.7 to 8.9. As the pH approaches the pKa of the anesthetic, the nonionized percentage increases, and so does the speed of onset. For example, lidocaine has a pKa of 7.9. At a pH of 4.5, such as that in commercial preparations containing epinephrine, only 3% is in the nonionized form. As the solution is buffered and approaches the pKa, the lipid-soluble fraction rises and increases the speed of onset. Conversely, injection into an acidotic area, such as that created by infection or inflammation, results in delayed onset of anesthesia.

Neural Stimulation

Local anesthetics inhibit depolarization by binding to voltage-gated Na^+ channels. Na^+ channels exist in constant transition between three states: closed (closed but can be opened by stimulus), activated (open), and inactivated (in absolute refractory and cannot be opened by stimulus) (38). Local anesthetics bind preferentially to channels in the inactivated state, such as those that are present after the nerve has fired but before repolarization has occurred (39). As such, a given concentration of local anesthetic will have a greater effect on rapidly firing neurons than those at rest. Thus, rubbing the area after infiltrating anesthesia not only provides distracting stimulus and improves tissue distribution, but it can stimulate the cutaneous nerves and increase the speed of blockade (32).

Duration

Long-acting agents and limiting local perfusion can prolong the duration of anesthesia. An anesthetic's duration is directly affected by its protein-binding ability and rate of metabolism. For example, the long-acting anesthetic bupivacaine is 96% protein bound, where intermediate-acting lidocaine is 64% and short-acting procaine 6% (40). Lidocaine is metabolized by cytochrome 3A4 of the P450 isoenzyme system. Patients taking medications that induce this isoenzyme, such as carbamazepine, dexamethasone, phenobarbital, and phenytoin, will have more rapid degradation of lidocaine and abbreviated anesthesia (41).

Highly perfused areas, such as the face, have shortened duration of anesthesia because of "vascular washout." To counteract this effect, most anesthetics are available with epinephrine. Epinephrine is a vasoconstrictor that when combined with an anesthetic decreases local perfusion and prolongs the duration of anesthesia. It also decreases intraoperative bleeding that may limit visualization of the operative field.

Diffusion

Diffusion of an anesthetic into surrounding tissue can be hastened by subcutaneous infiltration followed by massage of the area. Another method to enhance dispersion is to add hyaluronidase to the local anesthetic solution (Table 2). Hyaluronidase ezymatically digests the hyaluronic acid that is found in the intercellular ground substance of connective tissue. When added to a local anesthetic, it increases tissue permeability, allowing greater spread of anesthesia with less tissue distortion. It has also been noted to facilitate undermining in the subcutaneous plane and improves visualization of skin contours. Drawbacks are that it tends to decrease the duration of anesthesia, increases postoperative bruising, and has the potential to cause anaphylaxis (42). Commercial hyaluronidase (Vitrase® ISTA Pharmaceuticals, Irvine, California, U.S.) is bovine in origin and while anaphylaxis is rare, a skin test is recommended prior to use. According to the package insert, this consists of injecting 3 IU of reconstituted hyaluronidase and observing the site for development of a wheal with pseudopods that persists for 20 to 30 minutes.

TECHNIQUE

Universal Precautions

Infiltrating anesthesia into the skin is an invasive procedure that exposes the surgeon to potential bloodborne pathogens, and universal precautions should always apply. Protective measures include wearing gloves for all procedures, and since it is not unusual for the anesthetic to spray out of the skin during infiltration, eye protection should also be worn. A Luer-Lok syringe that secures the needle to its tip can limit its risk of popping off during infiltration into resistant tissue such as a keloid. The majority of needle stick injuries occur during recapping of a needle. This practice can be avoided by discarding the needle and syringe as a single unit immediately after injection. If recapping is necessary, the risk for needle stick can be reduced by using specially designed safety needles and syringe systems (43).

Drawing Up Anesthesia

The opening of a multidose vial is protected with a rubber stopper or membrane. This allows introduction of the needle to withdraw the fluid and closes tightly after the needle is removed. The surface is not sterile and must be wiped with alcohol prior to each insertion of the needle. To reduce vacuum formation, a small volume of air should be introduced into the bottle before aspirating into the syringe. It is more efficient to use a large-bore needle such as an 18 gauge that allows rapid fluid withdrawal. Once a sufficient amount of anesthetic is drawn into the syringe, the needle should be discarded in an appropriate container and exchanged for a 28- or 30-gauge needle. If additional anesthetic is needed during the procedure, a new syringe and needle should be used to withdraw it from the bottle (44). This practice eliminates the potential for cross-contamination.

Skin Preparation

Infiltration of anesthesia usually causes blanching and some degree of tumescence, which may limit the visualization or palpation of the lesion and distort surgical margins (18). This concern can be avoided by outlining the lesion with

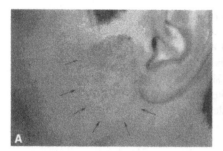 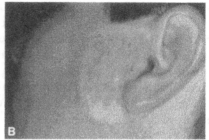

Figure 3 (**A**) Preoperative appearance of an infiltrative basal cell carcinoma with subtle peripheral margins (*black arrows*). (**B**) Appearance after infiltration of 1% lidocaine with epinephrine 1:200,000. Note: The inferior margins would be difficult to discern if they had not been marked preoperatively with gentian violet.

surgical ink, such as gentian violet, before infiltrating anesthesia (Fig. 3). To ensure accurate margins, such as for melanoma excision, the margins should be measured and outlined prior to infiltration.

Alcohol is an excellent agent to cleanse the skin before infiltration of an anesthetic. It has nearly instantaneous onset of action and very broad spectrum. However, it does not have any detergent qualities, and visible dirt or debris must be removed first with soap. Alternatives to alcohol include chlorhexidine gluconate and povidone-iodine. These agents have a similar spectrum but may take a few minutes to reach maximum effectiveness. They also tend to make the surface slippery and may limit the ability to grasp the tissue and stabilize it during infiltration.

Direct Infiltration

Direct infiltration is the most straightforward form of local anesthesia and is ideal for small skin biopsies or scissor excisions. The portion of skin to be sampled is cleansed with alcohol, and the anesthetic is infiltrated slowly into the tissue directly below the lesion. Superficial infiltration should be limited because it is more painful than deep dermal infiltration and can produce unwanted tumescence. A shave biopsy that was meant to be flush with the level of the surrounding skin may create a divot if the biopsy is performed on tumescent tissue. If there is concern that this may occur, the area can be massaged to help distribute the fluid before the biopsy is performed.

For open wounds, such as defects from Mohs micrographic surgery, it is less painful to inject through the wound rather than into the surrounding skin. Dripping the anesthetic solution into the wound can create a degree of topical anesthesia and decrease the pain from the needle stick. For clean defects, the anesthetic is infiltrated directly into the edges of the wound and extended in a radial fashion into the surrounding subcutaneous tissue. This technique is not appropriate for contaminated wounds, as it may encourage the spread of infection into the surrounding tissue.

Field Block

A field block achieves a larger area of anesthesia than direct infiltration below the lesion. It avoids infiltration into inflamed or infected tissue, which may be difficult to anesthetize directly. Infiltrating directly into a cyst, which may cause rupture, can be avoided by encircling it with a ring of anesthesia. Another use for a field block is when tumescence may limit the ability to palpate a subtle subcutaneous lesion that does not have appreciable epidermal change.

After the skin is cleansed with alcohol, the proposed surgical margins are marked with gentian violet. If the majority of the sensory innervation to that portion of the skin is unidirectional, then the first point of infiltration should be proximal and extend distally (Fig. 4). A 1-inch needle allows for a larger area to be anesthetized with a single needle stick and may be preferable for large fields. To anesthetize the surface, a small amount of anesthetic should be infiltrated superficially to raise a wheal (Fig. 5). Next, the needle is introduced through this wheal into the subcutaneous tissue. Prior to infiltration in the subcutaneous tissue, the surgeon should aspirate to evaluate for intravascular placement of the

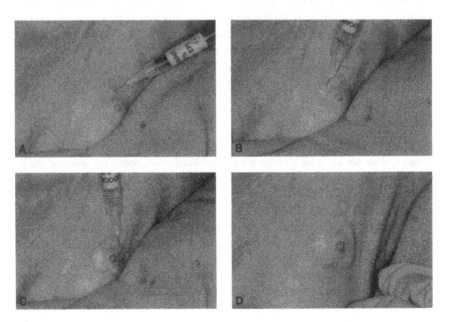

Figure 4 A 2-cm fluctuant cyst on the neck where rupture from infiltration of an anesthetic is particularly undesirable. (**A**) A small wheal is created. (**B–D**) The needle is introduced through the wheal and advanced through anesthetized skin to encircle the lesion without infiltrating directly into the cyst.

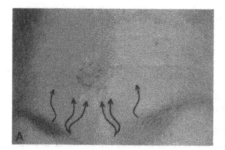 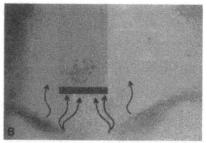

Figure 5 (**A**) Sensory innervation to the central forehead is largely derived from branches of the supratrochlear and supraorbital nerves that curve upward over the medial supraorbital rim and proceed superiorly (*arrows*). (**B**) Infiltration of a horizontal line of anesthetic across the nerves' path (*bar*) will provide distal anesthesia (*shaded zone*) and should be the first point of injection.

needle. It is important to remember that aspirating through a 30-gauge needle cannot reliably exclude intravascular placement, as the bore of the needle is too small to aspirate blood. A comprehensive understanding of anatomy and keeping the needle in motion during infiltration can reduce the risk for intravascular injection of large amounts of anesthetic. Once appropriate placement has been confirmed, the anesthetic is infiltrated slowly as the needle is advanced parallel to the surgical margin. To avoid breakage, the needle should not be inserted beyond two-thirds of its length (45). It is then withdrawn and reinserted into the skin that was anesthetized by the first infiltration. This is repeated sequentially until the entire circumference of the field has been anesthetized.

Scalp Block

There are several nerves that supply sensation to the scalp. The supraorbital and supratrochlear nerves, which innervate the forehead, also supply the anterior scalp. The zygomaticotemporal, auriculotemporal, and lesser occipital nerves supply the parietal portion and innervation to the occipital scalp is through the greater occipital and third occipital nerves. These sensory nerves extend in a superior direction, and a ring of anesthesia that begins at the level of the eyebrows continues across the superior auricular sulcus toward the occiput and back around to the starting point will anesthetize the entire scalp above it (46). This path crosses several large blood vessels such as the temporal artery; care must be taken to avoid intravascular injection or laceration of the artery with the bevel of the needle.

Ear Block

Infiltration of anesthesia around the base of the ear anesthetizes the auriculotemporal branch of the trigeminal nerve (V3), the greater auricular (C2, C3), and lesser occipital (C2, C3) nerves. This blocks the sensation of the external ear, with the exception of the conchal bowl, external auditory canal, and postauricular sulcus. These regions are supplied by branches of cranial nerves VII, IX, and X and must be injected directly to obtain reliable anesthesia. To perform this block, the needle is inserted at the inferior auricular sulcus, near the attachment of the lobe. Anesthetic is infiltrated anterosuperiorly toward the tragus in the subcutaneous plane. The needle is then withdrawn and redirected posterosuperiorly along the postauricular sulcus. Anesthetic is sequentially infiltrated toward and across the superior auricular sulcus. Next, the needle is placed at the tragus and the anesthetic is infiltrated superiorly along the preauricular sulcus to completely encircle the ear. Branches of the temporal artery lie within the path of infiltration, and care must be taken to avoid them. Lastly, the concha and external auditory canal must be anesthetized directly to complete the block.

Nose Block

The innervation to the nose is similar to the ear in that circumferential infiltration of anesthesia blocks sensory input to all but its central portion. Branches of the infraorbital nerve supply the lateral nose and inferior nasal ala, and the infratrochlear nerve innervates the superior portion. The nasal tip and columella receive input from the external nasal branches of the anterior ethmoidal nerve, which exit at the junction of the nasal bone and lateral cartilages. The first step in this block is to infiltrate within the alar sulcus extending superiorly along the nasofacial crease (Fig. 6). The needle is then redirected inferomedially, and anesthesia is infiltrated along the nostril sill to the columella, extending over the anterior nasal spine. This procedure is subsequently repeated on the opposite side. Next, the needle is placed midline at the junction of the dorsum and root of the nose. Anesthetic is infiltrated laterally toward the medial canthus and then inferiorly within the nasofacial crease on both sides. This ring of anesthesia encircles the nose and anesthetizes the entire cutaneous surface except for the tip, which is supplied by the anterior ethmoidal nerve. This nerve emerges at the distal edge of the nasal bone where it joins the upper lateral cartilages. Once this junction has been palpated, the needle is inserted in the midline and anesthesia is infiltrated bilaterally in inferolateral directions toward both sides of the nose to complete the block.

LOCAL EFFECTS OF ANESTHESIA

Blanching

As stated previously, epinephrine is frequently added to local anesthetic solutions to decrease bleeding and increase the duration of anesthesia (18). It also creates transient blanching from vasoconstriction that may be dramatic in patients with ruddy complexions. This usually lasts for 30 to 60 minutes but can be alarming if the patient is not reassured that it is expected and transient.

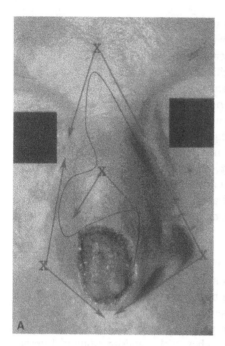 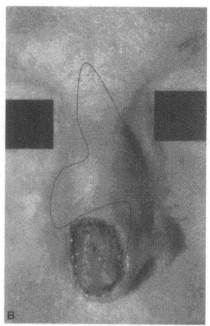

Figure 6 Nose block to achieve sufficient anesthesia for the (**A**) planned bilobed flap repair (*outlined in black*). (**B**) Injection points marked with an "X" and black arrows indicate the direction of infiltration.

Epinephrine can also limit the ability to discern the margins of ill-defined lesions. This can be avoided by outlining the lesion with surgical ink before infiltration of anesthesia.

Epinephrine vasoconstriction does not appear to impact the survival of undelayed local skin flaps, but it may have an adverse effect on full-thickness skin grafts (47,48). Fazio and Zitelli found that when lidocaine with epinephrine 1:200,000 was infiltrated into the donor site, there was a slightly increased risk of developing small areas of partial graft failure or epidermal necrosis at one week when compared with the plain lidocaine group (49). However, there was no correlation between epidermal necrosis, partial graft failure at one week, or the observed overall cosmetic outcome at six weeks. They hypothesized that the deleterious effect could have been due to prolonged vasoconstriction from delayed vascular inoculation and/or a direct harmful effect of epinephrine on the survival of vascular endothelial cells. Their conclusion was that since there was only minimal effect at one week and no effect on the six-week overall cosmetic outcome, there is no indication to harvest all full-thickness skin grafts with plain lidocaine. For wounds with compromised blood flow or oxygenation, such as in heavy smokers or poorly vascularized recipient sites, there may be a potential advantage to using plain lidocaine at the donor site.

Antibacterial Activity

The antibacterial effects of lidocaine were described in 1955 (50). Subsequent studies have confirmed that these effects are due to intrinsic antibacterial properties of lidocaine and not to methylparaben preservative. While the exact mechanism is not clear, the antibacterial effect tends to be pH dependent. When compared with plain lidocaine (pH 6.9), lidocaine with epinephrine (pH 4.5) has a less pronounced antibacterial effect (51). However, buffering lidocaine with epinephrine 1:10 with sodium bicarbonate (pH 7.4) dramatically increases its antibacterial properties beyond that of unbuffered plain lidocaine (52). The antibacterial spectrum includes *Staphylococcus aureus*, *Streptococcus pyogenes*, and gram-negative organisms such as *Escherichia coli*, *Klebsiella pneumoniae*, *Proteus mirabilis*, and *Pseudomona aeruginosa* (52,53). Animal studies have confirmed lidocaine's in vivo action against *S. aureus*, where wound infection did not occur despite deliberate innoculation (54).

Wound Healing

There is conflicting data regarding the effects of local anesthetics on wound healing. Morris and Tracey found a statistically significant, dose-dependent reduction of tensile strength in wounds infiltrated with lidocaine (55). This effect is partially due to injury from infiltration, since saline infiltration created the same reduction in tensile strength as 0.5% lidocaine. Upon review, the majority of studies tend to indicate that lidocaine may affect the first two phases of wound healing: inflammation and granulation/proliferation (56). However, this inhibition is both time and concentration dependent and would seem to apply to perfusion through a catheter and not to limited local infiltration.

COMPLICATIONS

Vasovagal Reaction

By far the most common complication from infiltrative anesthesia is a vasovagal reaction secondary to patient anxiety. This reaction manifests as nausea, diaphoresis, hyperventilation, bradycardia, and hypotension. If unchecked, it may progress to loss of consciousness. Vasovagal reactions can be distinguished from anaphylaxis by lack of peripheral vasodilation, tachycardia, or stridor. The most important component of managing vasovagal reactions is their prevention. Overly anxious patients or those with history of previous syncopal episodes may benefit from a preoperative anxiolytic. All procedures should be performed with the patient in the recumbent position. If the patients show signs of a vasovagal reaction, they should be placed in the Trendelenburg position immediately and a cool cloth applied to their head. Should this progress to loss of consciousness; spirits of ammonia may be helpful in reviving the patient. Although intravenous fluids are rarely needed in this condition, supplemental oxygen may be helpful.

Bleeding

Infiltration of anesthesia frequently causes ecchymosis that may be exaggerated in patients taking anticoagulants. They should be warned of this possibility during their postoperative instruction so that they are not alarmed should it occur. The bevel of the needle is sharp and may inadvertently cause injury to blood vessels, thus creating a hematoma. If this occurs, direct pressure without release should be applied for 20 minutes. The site should be observed for rebleeding and should this occur, pressure should be reapplied for an additional 20 minutes. Ice may also be of value if pressure alone should fail.

Edema

Local anesthetics are suspended in an isotonic solution that can create immediate tumescence followed by delayed edema from fluid redistribution. This is particularly true around the eyelids and lips, which are distended easily even when they are not infiltrated directly. For example, infiltration of anesthetic into the forehead or nose frequently causes extensive edema of the eyelids due to gravity. This can be limited by instructing patients to keep their head elevated as much as possible and to sleep on extra pillows. Cool compresses may also help relieve the swelling.

Infection

Infection may occur if close attention is not paid to appropriate aseptic technique. The outer surface of the anesthetic bottle should be cleaned with alcohol prior to each puncture of the needle, and the skin should be similarly cleansed before infiltrating anesthetic. Direct infiltration into a visibly purulent lesion or a contaminated wound should be avoided. In these cases, a field block or regional nerve block should be performed.

Nerve Laceration

Sensory nerve injury is usually manifested by paresthesias that may take several months to resolve. The risk for nerve injury is greatest with regional anesthesia but may also occur during local infiltration. If the needle punctures the nerve and anesthetic is infiltrated, the resulting hydrostatic pressure can create a compartment syndrome within the epineurium causing axolysis (40). In addition, the bevel of the needle is very sharp and can lacerate a nerve. Given its small diameter, permanent nerve damage from a 30-gauge needle is unlikely but certain precautions are still advised. Anesthetic should never be injected purposefully into a nerve or foramen. If the patient complains of an "electric" sensation, the needle should be withdrawn slightly until the paresthesias resolve, taking care to avoid any lateral motion.

REFERENCES

1. Wood A. New method of treating neuralgia by the direct application of opiates to the painful points. Edin Med Surg J 1855; 82:265–281.
2. Howard-Jones N. A critical study of the origins and early development of hypodermic medication. J Hist Med 1947; 2:201–249.
3. Lafargue GV. Lettre de M. le Docteur Lafargue de Saint-Emilion, sur l'inoculation de la morphine avec la lancette. Bull Acad Med Paris 1836; 1:13–18, 40–42.
4. Hunter C. Practical remarks on the hypodermical treatment of disease. Lancet 1863; 2:444–445, 675–676.
5. Lafitte L. Des injections sous-cutanées d'eau distillées ou d'eau pure; —leur bons effets thérapeutiques. L'Union médicale 1875; 20:445–448, 458–461.
6. Niemann A. Uber eine neue organische Base in den Cocablattern. Arch Pharm 1860; 153:129–155; 291–308.
7. Van Dyke C, Byck R. Cocaine. Sci Am 1982; 246:128–141.
8. Cobo B. Historia del nuevo mundo volume I. Sevilla: La Sociedad de Biliofilos Andaluces, 1890 [1653].
9. Koller K. Ueber die Verwendung des Cocain zur Aanasthesirung am Auge. Wien Med Wochenschr 1884; 34:1276–1278.
10. Koller C. Historical notes on the beginning of local anesthesia. J Am Med Assoc 1928; 90:1742–1743.
11. Halsted WS. Surgical papers by William Stewart Halsted (2 vol). Vol 1. Baltimore: The Johns Hopkins Press, 1922.
12. Schorr MR. Needles. Some points to think about. 1. Anesth Analg 1966; 45:509–513 contd.
13. Olch PD. William S. Halsted and local anesthesia: contributions and complications. Anesthesiology 1975; 42:479–486.
14. Goerig M. Carl Ludwig Schleich and the introduction of infiltration anesthesia into clinical practice. Reg Anesth Pain Med 1998; 23:538–539.
15. Goerig M, Bohrer H. [Historical vignette (6). Carl Ludwig Schleich and the scandal at the Berlin 1892 Surgical Congress]. Anasthesiol Intensivmed Notfallmed Schmerzther 1992; 27:453–454.
16. Bier A. Carl Ludwig Schleich. Zentralbl Chir 1922; 19:665–666.
17. Schooff M. Lessening the pain of lidocaine injection. J Fam Pract 1998; 46:279.
18. Grekin RC, Auletta MJ. Local anesthesia in dermatologic surgery. J Am Acad Dermatol 1988; 19:599–614.
19. Brogan GX Jr., Giarrusso E, Hollander JE, et al. Comparison of plain, warmed, and buffered lidocaine for anesthesia of traumatic wounds. Ann Emerg Med 1995; 26:121–125.
20. Woodfin CB. Warming bupivacaine for intradermal anesthesia. J Fam Pract 1998; 46:457.
21. Lugo-Janer G, Padial M, Sanchez JL. Less painful alternatives for local anesthesia. J Dermatol Surg Oncol 1993; 19:237–240.
22. Mader TJ, Playe SJ, Garb JL. Reducing the pain of local anesthetic infiltration: warming and buffering have a synergistic effect. Ann Emerg Med 1994; 23:550–554.
23. Robinson J, Fernando R, Sun Wai WY, et al. Chemical stability of bupivacaine, lidocaine and epinephrine in pH-adjusted solutions. Anaesthesia 2000; 55:853–858.

24. Stewart JH, Chinn SE, Cole GW, et al. Neutralized lidocaine with epinephrine for local anesthesia—II. J Dermatol Surg Oncol 1990; 16:842–845.
25. Howe NR, Williams JM. Pain of injection and duration of anesthesia for intradermal infiltration of lidocaine, bupivacaine, and etidocaine. J Dermatol Surg Oncol 1994; 20:459–464.
26. Xia Y, Chen E, Tibbits DL, et al. Comparison of effects of lidocaine hydrochloride, buffered lidocaine, diphenhydramine, and normal saline after intradermal injection. J Clin Anesth 2002; 14:339–343.
27. Green SM, Rothrock SG, Gorchynski J. Validation of diphenhydramine as a dermal local anesthetic. Ann Emerg Med 1994; 23:1284–1289.
28. Match DI. A pharmacological and therapeutic study of benzyl alcohol as a local anesthetic. J Pharmacol Exp Ther 1918; 11:263–279.
29. Holmes HS. Options for painless local anesthesia. Postgrad Med 1991; 89:71–72.
30. Swinehart JM. The ice-saline-xylocaine technique. A simple method for minimizing pain in obtaining local anesthesia. J Dermatol Surg Oncol 1992; 18:28–30.
31. Wiener SG. Injectable sodium chloride as a local anesthetic for skin surgery. Cutis 1979; 23:342–343.
32. Melzack R, Wall PD. Pain mechanisms: a new theory. Science 1965; 150:971–979.
33. Hodge B, Thompson JF. Noise pollution in the operating theatre. Lancet 1990; 335:891–894.
34. Whipple B, Glynn NJ. Quantification of the effects of listening to music as a non-invasive method of pain control. Sch Inq Nurs Pract 1992; 6:43–58; discussion 59–62.
35. Kim MS, Cho KS, Woo H, et al. Effects of hand massage on anxiety in cataract surgery using local anesthesia. J Cataract Refract Surg 2001; 27:884–890.
36. Moon JS, Cho KS. The effects of handholding on anxiety in cataract surgery patients under local anaesthesia. J Adv Nurs 2001; 35:407–415.
37. Fosko SW, Gibney MD, Harrison B. Repetitive pinching of the skin during lidocaine infiltration reduces patient discomfort. J Am Acad Dermatol 1998; 39:74–78.
38. Hodgkin AL, Huxley AF. A quantitative description of membrane current and its application to conduction and excitation in nerve. J Physiol 1952; 11:500–544.
39. Chen Z, Ong BH, Kambouris NG, et al. Lidocaine induces a slow inactivated state in rat skeletal muscle sodium channels. J Physiol 2000; 524(pt 1):37–49.
40. Schecter WP, Swisher JL. Local anesthesia in surgical practice. Curr Probl Surg 2000; 37:10–67.
41. Michalets EL. Update: clinically significant cytochrome P-450 drug interactions. Pharmacotherapy 1998; 18:84–112.
42. Clark LE, Mellette JR Jr. The use of hyaluronidase as an adjunct to surgical procedures. J Dermatol Surg Oncol 1994; 20:842–844.
43. Tomkins DP, van der Walt JH. Needleless and sharp-free anaesthesia. Anaesth Intensive Care 1996; 24:164–168.
44. Plott RT, Wagner RF Jr., Tyring SK. Iatrogenic contamination of multidose vials in simulated use. A reassessment of current patient injection technique. Arch Dermatol 1990; 126:1441–1444.
45. Smith DW, Peterson MR, DeBerard SC. Local anesthesia. Topical application, local infiltration, and field block. Postgrad Med 1999; 106:57–60, 64–66.
46. Seager DJ, Simmons C. Local anesthesia in hair transplantation. Dermatol Surg 2002; 28:320–328.

47. Wu G, Calamel PM, Shedd DP. The hazards of injecting local anesthetic solutions with epinephrine into flaps: experimental study. Plast Reconstr Surg 1978; 62: 396–403.
48. Wolfort S, Rohrich RJ, Handren J, et al. The effect of epinephrine in local anesthesia on the survival of full- and split-thickness skin grafts: an experimental study. Plast Reconstr Surg 1990; 86:535–540.
49. Fazio MJ, Zitelli JA. Full-thickness skin grafts. Clinical observations on the impact of using epinephrine in local anesthesia of the donor site. Arch Dermatol 1995; 131:691–694.
50. Murphy JT, Allen HF, Mangiaracine AB. Preparation, sterilization and preservation of ophthalmic solutions. AMA Arch Ophthalmol 1955; 53:63–78.
51. Barker W, Rodeheaver GT, Edgerton MT, et al. Damage to tissue defenses by a topical anesthetic agent. Ann Emerg Med 1982; 11:307–310.
52. Thompson KD, Welykyj S, Massa MC. Antibacterial activity of lidocaine in combination with a bicarbonate buffer. J Dermatol Surg Oncol 1993; 19:216–220.
53. Parr AM, Zoutman DE, Davidson JS. Antimicrobial activity of lidocaine against bacteria associated with nosocomial wound infection. Ann Plast Surg 1999; 43: 239–245.
54. Stratford AF, Zoutman DE, Davidson JS. Effect of lidocaine and epinephrine on *Staphylococcus aureus* in a guinea pig model of surgical wound infection. Plast Reconstr Surg 2002; 110:1275–1279.
55. Morris T, Tracey J. Lignocaine: its effects on wound healing. Br J Surg 1977; 64:902–903.
56. Brower MC, Johnson ME. Adverse effects of local anesthetic infiltration on wound healing. Reg Anesth Pain Med 2003; 28:233–240.

5

Regional Anesthesia

Conway C. Huang

*Department of Dermatology, University
of Alabama at Birmingham, Birmingham,
Alabama, U.S.A.*

INTRODUCTION

Nerve blocks involve injecting an anesthetic solution at the proximal aspect of a sensory nerve before it has significantly arborized for the purpose of obtaining widespread distal anesthesia. Competency in performing nerve blocks requires sound knowledge of suitable anesthetic agents and sensory nerve anatomy. The ability to reproducibly block key sensory nerves is valuable to physicians who perform surgical procedures under local anesthesia. This chapter will discuss advantages and disadvantages of nerve blocks, suitable anesthetic agents, and practical nerve blocks of the head and neck, wrist, ankle, and digits.

ADVANTAGES AND DISADVANTAGES OF NERVE BLOCKS OVER LOCAL INFILTRATION OF ANESTHESIA (1)

Advantages

- Nerve blocks can be less painful especially when dealing with the face, hands, and feet. For example, for anesthesia of the palm, it is generally less painful to block the median nerve at the proximal wrist flexion crease than to inject local anesthetic directly into the palm.

- Nerve blocks generally require a smaller volume of anesthetic since the injection is performed at a proximal location along the nerve before it has significantly arborized.
- Nerve blocks can generally anesthetize a wide, large area with a minimum of anesthetic dosage and number of injections. Blocks are ideally suited for achieving anesthesia in areas such as the palms and soles where wide local infiltration is nearly intolerable.
- Nerve blocks can be used in contaminated wounds where local infiltration may propagate infection.
- Nerve blocks result in almost no distortion of tissue compared to local infiltration. This is due to a combination of requiring less volume of anesthesia and performing the injections proximal to and distant from the operative/procedural field. This is helpful when distortion would interfere with fine tissue apposition (e.g., earlobe repair or facial laceration) or when excising subtle subcutaneous lesions (e.g., small epidermoid cysts or lipomas) where distortion of tissue might impede palpation and localization of the lesion.

Disadvantages and General Rules To Follow (2)

- There is a significant waiting time to allow for diffusion of the anesthetic into the nerve trunk. Depending on the area, this can take 30 minutes. *Allow sufficient time for diffusion of anesthetic into the nerve trunk.*
- There can be trauma to the neurovascular bundle by inadvertent needle laceration of the target nerve or its associated vessel. Trauma can also occur by intraneuronal injection causing volume tamponade that can lead to temporary neuropraxia or even permanent nerve damage. Paresthesias or severe pain during injection is a sign that neuronal laceration or intraneuronal injection may be occurring. *If one of these signs is encountered, immediately cease injection, reposition the needle (usually more superficially), and resume injection.* Inadvertent intra-arterial injection can lead to hematoma and/or unwanted systemic side effects. *Aspirating before injecting in areas with named arteries and repositioning the needle tip frequently during injection are techniques that can minimize the risk of intra-arterial injection.*
- Anesthetic overdosing can occur since many physicians use 2% lidocaine to aid in penetration of the nerve sheath. Obviously, one is limited to half the volume of 1% lidocaine and must keep this in mind especially when performing multiple blocks (e.g., multiple digital blocks). *Always consider volume and dosing limitations.*

ANESTHETIC AGENTS

One percent or 2% lidocaine without epinephrine is the primary anesthetic used for nerve blocks. Selecting which concentration of lidocaine to use depends on several factors including the patient's weight and the volume of anesthetic

Table 1 Lidocaine Dosing

Anesthetic agent	Maximum recommended dose (mg/kg)
Lidocaine	4.5
Lidocaine with epinephrine	7.0

needed to perform the necessary nerve block(s). One percent lidocaine contains 10 mg/cc of lidocaine. Two percent contains 20 mg/cc. For a 50-kg patient, one can inject 225 mg of lidocaine without epinephrine (Table 1). This equates to 22.5 cc of 1% lidocaine without epinephrine or 11.2 cc of 2% lidocaine without epinephrine. If one were to perform nerve blocks on five fingers, it would be easier to use 1% lidocaine where 4.5 cc (22.5 cc/5 fingers) could be used per finger. While 2% lidocaine would theoretically be more effective at penetrating nerve sheath, only 2.2 cc per finger would be available at that concentration. This lesser volume potentially negates any nerve sheath diffusion advantage that would be obtained from the higher concentration of lidocaine. Therefore, since one can use twice the volume of anesthetic of 1% lidocaine compared to 2%, 1% is more suited for a low body weight patient who needs multiple blocks or blocks that require larger volumes of anesthesia. Two percent lidocaine is better suited for patients who can receive higher doses of lidocaine (heavier weight) and/or who have limited areas that need nerve blocks. Before performing a nerve block, calculate dosing and/or volume limitations for the patient in question and select the most appropriate concentration.

It is dogma to exclude epinephrine especially in blocks involving areas of nonredundant blood supply such as the penis and digits. While there is scant evidence to support this, it represents the current standard of care. Recently, there is evidence to suggest that the use of epinephrine in nerve blocks is safe even in areas of nonredundant blood supply. The decision to use epinephrine is an individual one that should be made on a patient-by-patient basis (3–7).

Other anesthetic agents are not discussed here due to the extreme rarity of true allergic reaction to lidocaine and to the overwhelming prevalence of the use of lidocaine for nerve blocks. In the rare instance that lidocaine is contra-indicated, ester anesthetics or other agents such as normal saline preserved with benzyl alcohol or dilute benadryl can be used. A detailed discussion of these is beyond the scope of this chapter. The reader is referred to many excellent articles available with a simple literature search.

HEAD AND NECK BLOCKS (8–10)

Sensory innervation of the skin of the head and neck (H&N) is primarily derived from cranial nerve V (the trigeminal nerve) and several cervical nerves (greater auricular, auriculotemporal, and greater and lesser occipital nerves). The conchal

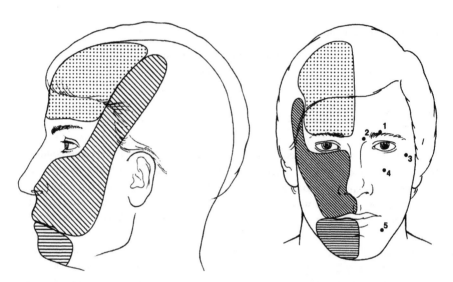

Figure 1 Facial sensory innervation; dotted area, V1; oblique lines, V2; horizontal lines, V3; 1, supraorbital notch (entry point of supraorbital nerve); 2, supratrochlear nerve entry point; 3, zygomaticotemporal nerve entry point; 4, infraorbital foramen (entry point of infraorbital nerve); 5, mental foramen (entry point of mental nerve).

bowl is supplied by sensory branches from cranial nerves 7, 9, and 10. From a practical standpoint, the H&N has been divided into the following areas: V1, V2, V3, nose, ear, and scalp (Fig. 1). Nerve blocks of each of these areas will be discussed individually.

V1

Area: Refer to Figure 1.

Potential uses: Anesthesia for chemical peels, dermabrasion, nonablative or ablative laser procedures, injection of filler substances, and/or incisional or excisional surgery. Note that with incisional or excisional surgery, supplemental local infiltration of anesthetic with epinephrine may be desirable for its added hemostatic effect.

Sensory nerve supply: Supratrochlear and supraorbital nerves (Fig. 1).

Nerve block technique(s) (Fig. 1):

1. Locate the supraorbital notch. This is palpable along the superior orbital rim in the midpupillary line.
2. Inject 2 to 3 mL of 1–2% lidocaine (choose concentration after considering volume and dosing limitations) in a fan-shaped pattern superior to the supraorbital notch. This will block the supraorbital nerve. Injection depth should be submuscular (deep to the corrugator) near the bony surface.

3. Directly medial to the supraorbital notch, along the superiomedial orbital rim, inject another 2 to 3 mL of anesthetic in a fan-shaped pattern as above. This will block the supratrochlear nerve.

V2

Area: Refer to Figure 1.

Potential uses: Anesthesia for chemical peels, dermabrasion, nonablative or ablative laser procedures, injection of filler substances, and/or incisional or excisional surgery. Note that with incisional or excisional surgery, supplemental local infiltration of anesthetic with epinephrine may be desirable for its added hemostatic effect.

Sensory nerve supply: Infraorbital and zygomaticotemporal nerves (Fig. 1).

Nerve block technique(s) (Fig. 1):

1. Identify the infraorbital foramen. This is located in the midpupillary line approximately 2 cm below the inferior orbital rim.
2. Inject 2 to 3 mL of 1–2% lidocaine (choose concentration after considering volume and dosing limitations) in a fan-shaped pattern circumferentially around the foramen. This will block the infraorbital nerve. Injection depth should be submuscular near the bony surface.
3. Along the zygoma, approximately 2 cm lateral to and 2 cm inferior to the lateral canthus, inject 2 to 3 mL of anesthetic in a fan-shaped pattern as above. This will block the zygomaticotemporal nerve. Injection should be submuscular near the bony surface.

V3

Area: Refer to Figure 1.

Potential uses: Anesthesia for chemical peels, dermabrasion, nonablative or ablative laser procedures, injection of filler substances, and/or incisional or excisional surgery. Note that with incisional or excisional surgery, supplemental local infiltration of anesthetic with epinephrine may be desirable for its added hemostatic effect.

Sensory nerve supply: Mental nerve (Fig. 1).

Nerve block technique(s) (Fig. 1):

1. Identify the mental foramen. This is located in the midpupillary line midway between the alveolar margin and the inferior border of the mandible.
2. Inject 2 to 3 mL of 1–2% lidocaine (choose concentration after considering volume and dosing limitations) in a fan-shaped pattern circumferentially around the foramen. This will block the mental nerve. Injection depth should be submuscular near the bony surface.

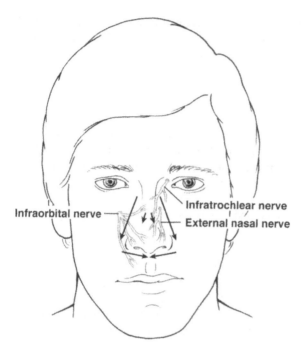

Figure 2   Technique for nasal sensory block.

Nose (8–10)

Area: Refer to Figure 2.

Potential uses: Anesthesia for chemical peels, dermabrasion, nonablative or ablative laser procedures, and/or incisional or excisional surgery. Note that with incisional or excisional surgery, supplemental local infiltration of anesthetic with epinephrine may be desirable for its added hemostatic effect.

Sensory nerve supply: Infratochlear, infraorbital, and anterior nasal nerves (Fig. 2).

Nerve block technique(s) (Fig. 2):

1. Starting at the nasal bridge, tunnel an injection into the deep subcutaneous fat with 1–2% lidocaine with or without epinephrine (choose concentration after considering volume and dosing limitations) extending inferiorly along either side of the nasal bone. Two mL of anesthetic per side should be sufficient. This will block the infratrochlear nerves.
2. Continue this tunnel of anesthesia inferiorly along each nasojugal sulcus until reaching the junction of the root of the nasal ala, the medial cheek, and the upper cutaneous lip. It will be less painful if subsequent injections are made into areas previously anesthetized by prior injections. Two mL of

anesthetic per side should be sufficient. This will block the medial fibers of the infraorbital nerve.

3. At this point, direct the tunnel of anesthesia directly medial along the border between the inferior rims of the nostrils and the upper cutaneous lip. Two mL of anesthetic per side should be sufficient. This will block medial fibers of the infraorbital and mental nerves.
4. Along the dorsal nose, locate the junction between the bony and cartilaginous nose. In the deep subcutaneous tissue, inject anesthetic along the dorsal and lateral aspects of the nose. Two mL of anesthetic per side should be sufficient. This will block the anterior nasal nerve.

Ear (8–10)

Area: Refer to Figure 3.

Potential uses: Anesthesia for chemical peels, nonablative or ablative laser procedures, and/or incisional or excisional surgery. Note that with incisional or excisional surgery, supplemental local infiltration of anesthetic with epinephrine may be desirable for its added hemostatic effect.

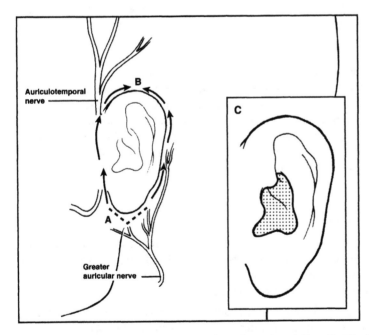

Figure 3 A, block of earlobe only—inject along dotted line; B, Block of entire ear excluding conchal bowl—inject along dotted line and solid line; C, conchal bowl—the dotted area is innervated by cranial nerves 7, 9, and 10 and is best anesthetized with local infiltration.

Sensory nerve supply: Greater auricular, auriculotemporal, and sensory portions of cranial nerves 7, 9, and 10 (Fig. 3).

Nerve block technique(s) (Fig. 3):

Earlobe only: Locate a point 2 to 3 cm directly inferior to the attachment of the earlobe. From this point, inject a tunnel of 1–2% lidocaine with or without epinephrine (choose concentration after considering volume and dosing limitations) in a V-shaped pattern into the deep subcutaneous fat. A total of 4 mL of anesthetic should be sufficient. This will block fibers of the greater auricular and auriculotemporal nerves supplying the earlobe. Note areas of the ear other than the lobe will likely have at least partial sensation.

Entire ear excluding conchal bowl:

1. Perform the injection for the earlobe as above.
2. Continue this injection upward along the anterior and posterior attachments of the pinna. At the superior attachment of the ear (crus of helix), the injections should wrap around and meet directly over the superior curve of the helix. Approximately 10 mL of anesthetic should suffice for this entire injection. This injection pattern will block fibers of the greater auricular and auriculotemporal nerves.

Conchal bowl: Due to its relatively small surface area and its separate innervation by cranial nerves 7, 9, and 10, local infiltration is the most effective technique to anesthetize this area. Two to three mL of 1–2% lidocaine with epinephrine (choose concentration after considering volume and dosing limitations) should be injected into the superficial subcutaneous space. This will block sensory fibers of cranial nerves 7, 9, and 10.

Scalp (8–10)

Area: Refer to Figure 4.

Potential uses: Anesthesia for chemical peels, dermabrasion, nonablative or ablative laser procedures, and/or incisional or excisional surgery. Note that with incisional or excisional surgery, supplemental local infiltration of anesthetic with epinephrine may be desirable for its added hemostatic effect.

Sensory nerve supply: Supratrochlear, supraorbital, zygomaticotemporal, auriculotemporal, greater auricular, greater and lesser occipital (Fig. 4).

Nerve block technique(s) (Fig. 4): Injections are tailored according to the area(s) of the scalp that require anesthesia.

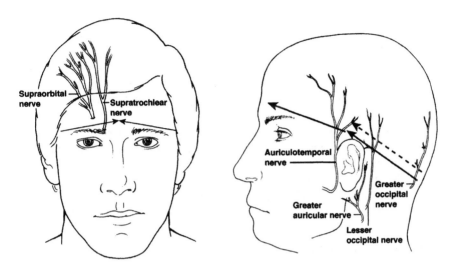

Figure 4 A, block frontal scalp—inject along thin arrows (frontal view); B, block parietal scalp—inject along thick arrows (side view); C, block occipital scalp—inject along dotted arrows (side view); D, block entire scalp—inject along A, B, and C as described above.

Frontal scalp and corresponding frontal areas of the vertex scalp: The supratrochlear and supraorbital nerves must be blocked for anesthesia of these areas. Injections should be performed as for V1 (refer to the section above). Block one or both sides depending on the where anesthesia is needed. Note that anesthesia of the corresponding forehead will also be obtained.

Parietal scalp and corresponding parietal areas of the vertex scalp: The zygomaticotemporal, auriculotemporal, and greater auricular nerves must be blocked for anesthesia of these areas. A tunnel of 1–2% lidocaine with or without epinephrine (choose concentration after considering volume and dosing limitations) should be injected into the deep subcutaneous fat extending from the lateral brow to a point 1 cm above the attachment of the crus of the helix. From that point, the injection should be continued to the midline of the nuchal crest. Anesthesia with epinephrine is recommended to prolong duration of effect. Without supplemental epinephrine, washout of anesthesia in the vascular scalp can occur sooner than desired. Block one or both sides depending on the where anesthesia is needed.

Occipital scalp and corresponding occipital areas of the vertex scalp: The greater and lesser occipital nerves must be blocked for anesthesia of these areas. A tunnel of 1–2% lidocaine with or without epinephrine (choose concentration after considering volume and dosing limitations) should be injected into the deep subcutaneous fat extending from 1 cm above the attachment of the crus of the helix to the midline of the nuchal crest. Anesthesia with epinephrine is recommended to prolong duration of effect. Without supplemental epinephrine, washout of anesthesia in the vascular scalp can occur sooner than desired. Block one or both sides depending on the where anesthesia is needed.

Entire scalp: To block the entire scalp, one would perform the above injections (frontal, parietal, and occipital scalp) in order. Note that the volume of anesthesia required to block the entire scalp can be large. In cases where one is confronted with volume and dosing limitations, 0.25–0.5% lidocaine can be used if needed. Anesthetic with epinephrine may be desirable for its added duration of effect.

WRIST BLOCKS (10–15)

There are three main areas of the hand upon which dermatologic surgeons perform procedures. These are the palmar surface, the dorsal hand, and the digits. Of these, the primary areas dermatologic surgeons have need of blocking are the palmar surface and the digits. The pain induced by local infiltration of anesthesia in these areas is nearly intolerable. On the other hand, the dorsal hand is supplied by the radial nerve, which can be blocked, but one can obtain equivalent, if not superior, anesthesia with local infiltration with the added hemostatic benefit of epinephrine. Local infiltration of anesthesia in the dorsal hand is minimally painful and is comparable to the pain associated with a radial nerve block. Therefore, this section will focus on blocks that anesthetize the palm and the digits.

Palm (11–16)

Area: Refer to Figure 5.

Potential uses: Anesthesia for injection of botulinum exotoxin or other substances into the palm for hyperhidrosis or other indications, nonablative or ablative laser procedures, and/or incisional or excisional surgery. Note that with incisional or excisional surgery, supplemental local infiltration of anesthetic with epinephrine may be desirable for its added hemostatic effect.

Sensory nerve supply: Median and ulnar nerves (Fig. 5).

Nerve block technique(s) (Fig. 6):

1. Locate the median nerve by asking the patient to form a fist and to flex at the wrist against resistance. The median nerve will course in between the easily visible palmaris longus and flexor carpi radialis tendons. Note that in <10% of patients, the palmaris longus tendon will be absent. In this case, use the flexor carpi radialis tendon as the ulnar landmark and the

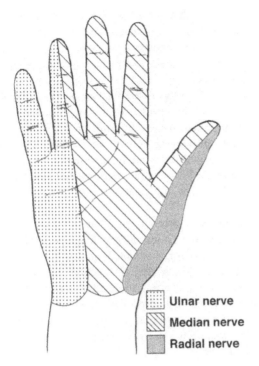

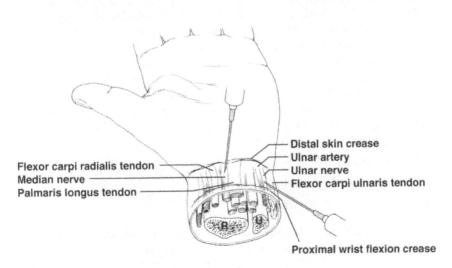

Figure 5 Neural innervation of the palm and digits.

Flexor carpi radialis tendon
Median nerve
Palmaris longus tendon

Distal skin crease
Ulnar artery
Ulnar nerve
Flexor carpi ulnaris tendon

Proximal wrist flexion crease

Figure 6 Nerve block technique for the median and ulnar nerves.

proximal aspect of the palmar "crease" that forms between the thenar and hypothenar eminences as the radial landmark to determine the course of the median nerve. The nerve will run in between these two landmarks. Note that the above mentioned "crease" can be accentuated by asking the patient to appose the thumb and ring finger.

2. The injection point will be along the course of the median nerve at the proximal wrist flexion crease. At this point, insert a 27 to 30 gauge needle approximately 2 cm perpendicularly, and inject 3 to 5 mL of 1–2% lidocaine (choose concentration after considering volume and dosing limitations) in a fan-shaped pattern. This will block the median nerve.

3. Locate the ulnar nerve by palpating the flexor carpi ulnaris tendon and the ulnar artery. The ulnar nerve will course immediately between the two structures.

4. The injection point will be along the course of the ulnar nerve at the proximal wrist flexion crease. At this point, insert a 27 to 30 gauge needle approximately 2 cm between the flexor carpi ulnaris tendon and the ulnar artery. Aspirate before injecting to avoid intra-arterial injection and inject 3 to 5 mL of 1–2% lidocaine (choose concentration after considering volume and dosing limitations) in a fan-shaped pattern. If blood is aspirated, withdraw the needle 2 to 3 mm, reposition it, and aspirate again. Repeat as needed to avoid intra-arterial injection. Apply pressure as needed. This will block the ulnar nerve.

Digits (Fingers) (11–16)

Note that there are two methods of blocking the digit that are used by the majority of dermatologic surgeons. These are the digital block and the "ring" block. The classic digital block involves bilateral injections at the surgical neck of the proximal phalanx near the metacarpophalangeal joint entering with a 2.5-cm 27- to 30-gauge needle from the dorsal hand, directing the needle toward the palmar subcutaneous tissue, and injecting 2 to 3 mL of 1–2% lidocaine (choose concentration after considering volume and dosing limitations) in a fan-shaped pattern. The "ring" block is much simpler conceptually and, in this author's opinion, results in more complete anesthesia more frequently. For these reasons, only this method will be discussed.

Area: Refer to Figure 7

Sensory nerve supply: Digital nerves (Fig. 7)

Nerve block technique(s) (Fig. 7):

1. Select the digit to be blocked. Identify the metacarpophalangeal joint. Identify the corresponding proximal interphalangeal joint. Each digit will have bilateral dorsal and palmar digital nerves that course along each lateral aspect of the proximal phalanx.

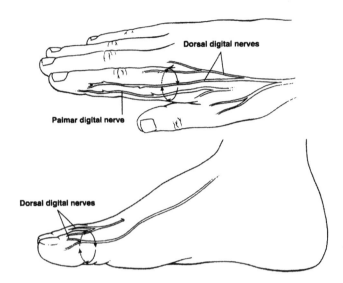

Figure 7 Ringed arrows indicate location of subcutaneous injections to achieve digital "ring" block.

2. The injection will occur along a path as if it were a "ring." The injection should be made into the subcutaneous fat. From there, anesthesia will diffuse to the deeper neurovascular bundle. One should not attempt to elicit paresthesia or to "step the needle" along the bony phalanx as this increases the risk of laceration of the neurovascular bundle and/or intraneuronal injection. Not more than 4 to 6 mL of 1–2% lidocaine (choose concentration after considering volume and dosing limitations) should be injected in order to avoid volume tamponade/compression of the neurovascular bundle. This injection will block the bilateral dorsal and palmar digital nerves.

Ankle Blocks (16–18)

There are three main areas of the foot upon which dermatologic surgeons perform procedures. These are the plantar surface, the dorsal foot, and the digits. Of these, the primary areas where dermatologic surgeons have need of blocking are the plantar surface and the digits. The pain induced by local infiltration of anesthesia in these areas is nearly intolerable. On the other hand, the dorsal foot is supplied by the superficial and deep peroneal and saphenous nerves, which can be blocked, but one can obtain equivalent, if not superior, anesthesia with local infiltration with the added hemostatic benefit of epinephrine. Local infiltration of anesthesia in the dorsal foot is minimally painful and is comparable to the pain associated with an anterior ankle (superficial and deep peroneal and saphenous nerves) nerve block. Therefore, this section will focus on blocks that anesthetize the plantar surface and the digits.

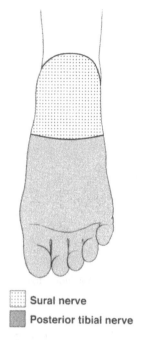

[ ] Sural nerve
[■] Posterior tibial nerve

Figure 8 Neural innervation of the sole and digits.

Sole (16–18)

Area: Refer to Figure 8.

Sensory nerve supply: Posterior tibial and sural nerves (Fig. 9).

Nerve block technique(s) (Fig. 9):

1. Place the patient in the prone position. Locate the posterior tibial nerve by drawing a line connecting the eminence of the medial malleolus and the midpoint of the arc of the posterior curve of the heel. Palpate the posterior tibial artery where it crosses this line. The nerve will course immediately posterior to the artery.
2. The injection point will be directly posterior to the posterior tibial artery. Advance the needle until encountering the underlying calcaneus. At this point, withdraw the needle 2 to 3 mm, aspirate, and, if no blood is aspirated, inject 3 to 5 mL of 1–2% lidocaine (choose concentration after considering volume and dosing limitations) in a fan-shaped pattern. If blood is aspirated, withdraw the needle 2 to 3 mm, reposition it, and aspirate again. Repeat as needed to avoid intra-arterial injection. Apply pressure as needed. This will block the posterior tibial artery.

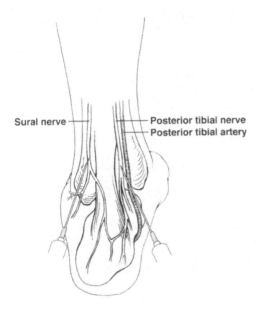

Sural nerve — Posterior tibial nerve
— Posterior tibial artery

Figure 9 Nerve block technique for sural and posterior tibial nerves.

3. Locate the sural nerve by identifying the eminence of the lateral malleolus and the Achilles tendon. The nerve courses along bone between these two landmarks.
4. The injection point will be between the eminence of the lateral malleolus and the Achilles tendon. In this area, advance the needle until the underlying bone is encountered, withdraw the needle 2 to 3 mm, and inject 3 to 5 mL of 1–2% lidocaine (choose concentration after considering volume and dosing limitations) in a fan-shaped pattern. This will block the sural nerve.

Digits (Toes) (16–18)

All aspects of nerve blocks for toes are identical to fingers [see section on "Digits (Fingers)"e].

REFERENCES

1. Quail G. Regional nerve blocks. Aust Fam Physician 1996; 25:1391–1396.
2. Smith DW, Peterson MR, DeBerard SC. Regional anesthesia. Nerve blocks of the extremities and face. Postgrad Med 1999; 106:68–78.
3. Altinyazar HC, Ozdemir H, Koca R, et al. Epinephrine in digital block: color doppler flow imaging. Dermatol Surg 2004; 30:508–511.
4. Denkler K. A comprehensive review of epinephrine in the finger: to do or not to do. Plast Reconstr Surg 2001; 108:114–124.

5. Krunic AL, Wang LC, Soltani K, et al. Digital anesthesia with epinephrine: an old myth revisited. J Am Acad Dermatol 2004; 51:755–759.

6. Wilhelmi BJ, Blackwell SJ, Miller J, et al. Epinephrine in digital blocks: revisited. Ann Plast Surg 1998; 41:410–414.

7. Wilhelmi BJ, Blackwell SJ, Miller JH et al. Do not use epinephrine in digital blocks: myth or truth? Plast Reconstr Surg 2001; 107:393–397.

8. Simpson S. Regional nerve blocks. Part 3-Regional blocks of the hand. Aust Fam Physician 2001; 7:669–671.

9. Zide BM, Swift R. How to block and tackle the face. Plast Reconstr Surg 1998; 101:840–850.

10. Eaton JS, Grekin RC. Regional anesthesia of the face. Dermatol Surg 2001; 27: 1006–1009.

11. Simpson S. Regional nerve blocks. Part 2-The face and scalp. Aust Fam Physician 2001; 30:565–568.

12. Fujita M, Mann T, Mann O, et al. Surgical pearl: use of nerve blocks for botulinum toxin treatment of palmar-plantar hyperhidrosis. J Am Acad Dermatol 2001; 45: 587–589.

13. Thompson WL, Malchow RJ. Peripheral nerve blocks and anesthesia of the hand. Military Med 2002; 167:478–482.

14. Hayton MJ, Stanley JK, Lowe, NJ. A review of peripheral nerve blockade as local anesthesia in the treatment of palmar hyperhidrosis. Br J Dermatol 2003; 149:447–451.

15. Campanati A, Lagalla G, Penna L, et al. A. Local neural block at the wrist for tx of palmar hyperhid with BTA: technical improvements. J Am Acad Dermatol 2004; 51: 345–348.

16. Ferrera PC, Chandler R. Anesthesia in the emergency setting: Part I. Hand and foot injuries. Am Fam Physician 1994; 50:569–573.

17. Colgrove RC. Technique tip: posterior tibial nerve block. Foot Ankle Int 2001; 22: 839–840.

18. Hess J. A review of regional blocks of the foot. J Am Assoc Nurse Anesth 1998; 66:82–87.

6

Tumescent Anesthesia

William B. Henghold

*The Skin Cancer Center of NW Florida,
Pensacola, Florida, U.S.A.*

Brent R. Moody

*Vanderbilt University Medical Center, Nashville,
Tennessee, U.S.A.*

INTRODUCTION

Tumescent anesthesia (TA) is a distinct form of local anesthesia that employs a large volume of fluid (usually normal saline) containing a very dilute concentration of anesthetic (primarily lidocaine) and vasoconstrictor (epinephrine), as well as other additives (notably, sodium bicarbonate). Local anesthesia is defined as the loss of sensation within a confined area without alteration of the patient's consciousness. *Tumescent* is derived from the Latin word *tumescere,* meaning to swell. It is the swelling and resultant firmness of the tissue that both contributes to the regional anesthetic effect and also facilitates the procedure for which it is now most commonly employed, liposuction. TA is *local infiltration* anesthesia and should not be confused with *regional* anesthesia as occurs with peripheral nerve blockade.

Klein developed the tumescent technique in the 1980s as a way to improve both the safety and efficacy of liposuction surgery. Since its introduction, TA has been used for a variety of other surgical procedures and in many ways has revolutionized the practice of dermatologic surgery. Procedures that were once done only under general anesthesia or by sedation analgesia are now safely and routinely performed in an outpatient, office-based setting.

HISTORY

In 1986 Klein introduced the tumescent technique at the Second World Congress of Liposuction Surgery, and his work first appeared in the medical literature the following year (1,2). The technique grew out of Klein's burgeoning interest in liposuction and a concern over the safety of the procedure as it was then practiced. Strictly speaking, the tumescent "technique," as described by Klein, refers to the way liposuction is performed, i.e., TA and microcannular liposuction performed *without* any other form of anesthesia (general or conscious sedation) or intravenous (IV) fluids (1). The distinction is important, because significant morbidity and mortality have been linked to the tumescent technique (in particular, lidocaine toxicity) when in fact these bad outcomes were most likely the result of other factors, namely, IV fluid overload or the effects of general anesthesia (3–5). TA, referring only to that specific form of anesthesia and irrespective of the operation subsequently performed, has been termed in the literature the tumescent technique (6), tumescent anesthesia technique (TAT) (7), and tumescent technique anesthesia (TTA) (8). Interestingly, in one report on the treatment of burn patients, lidocaine was left out of the solution altogether, but it was still referred to as the tumescent technique. (9).

Prior to the introduction of the tumescent technique, liposuction cases were usually done in a hospital setting under general anesthesia. Significant surgical blood loss necessitating transfusion was the rule rather than the exception. There was some attempt made to minimize bleeding by first instilling a dilute concentration of epinephrine (the *wet technique*), but anesthesia was still provided to the patient by inhalational or IV means. It was thought that the amount of local anesthetic, primarily lidocaine, necessary to achieve adequate anesthesia for moderate-volume or large-volume liposuction surgery was far too great to be administered safely. At that time (and to this day), the U.S. Food and Drug Administration's (FDA) approved maximum safe lidocaine dosage for adults, as it is reported in the Physicians' Desk Reference (PDR), is 4.5 mg/kg of body weight (total dose not to exceed 300 mg or 30 mL of a 1% solution) for plain lidocaine and 7 mg/kg (total dose 500 mg or 50 mL) for 1% lidocaine with epinephrine (10). [Note that *dosage* (milligram of drug per kilogram of patient body weight) and *dose* (milligram of drug) are distinct terms.]

No human trials examining the maximum safe dose of lidocaine have been performed, and the vast majority of reports in the literature concerning lidocaine toxicity in humans have nothing to do with local infiltration into the skin and subcutaneous fat, but rather into highly vascular tissue or directly into the

Table 1 Factors Affecting Peak Plasma Concentrations of Lidocaine

Lidocaine concentration in anesthetic solution
Epinephrine concentration in anesthetic solution
Rate of anesthetic infiltration
Target tissue characteristics
    Vascularity
    Fat content
Tumescent effect
Drug interactions (affecting lidocaine metabolism)
Patient factors
    Age
    Sex
    Liver function
    Body habitus

vasculature (11). The 7-mg/kg dosage limit for lidocaine with epinephrine may be a conservative dose when applied to the tumescent technique.

A study done in 1948 on mice showed that the lethal dose of lidocaine was inversely proportional to its concentration (12). It took twice the dose of a 0.5% solution to reach the median lethal dose (LD50) compared with a 2% solution. From this study, it could be reasoned that the total safe dose for lidocaine is best viewed as a function of its concentration and not as an absolute number; therefore, what may be valid for a plain 1% solution (300 mg, as mentioned earlier) is certainly not for a 0.1% solution. Of course, pharmacologic principles tell us that the interplay of a host of factors affects the ultimate safe and effective dose of any drug. The addition of epinephrine to the tumescent solution, the compression of blood and lymphatic vessels due to the swelling of the tissue itself, the relative avascularity of the subcutaneous fat into which the solution is instilled, and the high degree of lipid solubility of lidocaine all slow down the absorption of the drug into the circulation, which allows the liver to metabolize it efficiently (Table 1).

With careful clinical observation and continuous refinement of the tumescent technique, Klein and others following his lead have proceeded to push the envelope with respect to the maximum safe dose for lidocaine delivered by the tumescent route. Lillis looked at serum lidocaine levels and blood loss using the tumescent technique for liposuction (13). Even with dosages averaging 61 mg/kg (range, 31–89 mg/kg), the peak serum lidocaine concentrations one hour after administration of TA remained well below toxic levels. Blood loss was negligible, with preoperative and one-week postoperative hematocrit levels virtually identical. Later studies showed that peak serum lidocaine levels actually occur anywhere from 4 to 14 hours after administration of the tumescent solution and support the observation that patients experience an anesthetic effect many hours after completion of the procedure (14–16). The tumescent technique's proven ability to enhance hemostasis and provide prolonged postoperative pain relief, all while achieving a level of anesthesia that obviates general or IV routes of administration, has led to its use in a wide variety of procedures. The development of TA is without question one of the most important advances in the practice of dermatologic surgery.

PHARMACOLOGY OF TA

The safe and effective use of any drug necessitates a thorough understanding of the pharmacodynamic and pharmacokinetic principles at work. Pharmacodynamics deals with the mechanism of action of a drug and the relationship between a drug's concentration and its effect, and pharmacokinetics deals with its absorption, distribution, biotransformation, and elimination (17). After medical school and before his dermatology residency, and in addition to an internal medicine residency and a master's degree in public health, Dr. Klein spent two years as a National Institutes of Health research fellow in clinical pharmacology. In this way, he was uniquely prepared to critically evaluate the entrenched, dogmatic practices of the time. In his seminal work, Klein challenged the 7-mg/kg dosage limitation for lidocaine with epinephrine (2). In 26 patients who underwent liposuction entirely under local anesthesia, a mean dosage of 18.4 mg/kg was achieved with no clinical signs of toxicity. But how was this possible? An understanding of the pharmacologic principles at work helps answer the question. TA takes advantage of the unique properties of several drugs and their interaction with each other and the target tissue, all of which contributes to the final desired result, safe and complete local anesthesia of a large region. Each component of the solution will be discussed in further detail.

Lidocaine

Since the arrival of the first local anesthetic, cocaine, the clinical utility and potential toxicity of anesthetic agents has been well documented. Niemann first isolated cocaine in 1860, and Koller first used it clinically for ophthalmologic procedures in 1884. The first synthetic local anesthetic was the ester derivative procaine, discovered by Einhorn in 1905. Lofgren synthesized the amide lidocaine in 1943. It was an improvement over procaine, producing faster, more reliable, and longer-lasting effects.

The chemical structure of most local anesthetic agents is similar. They consist of three components: a lipophilic and a hydrophilic portion separated by a connecting hydrocarbon chain (either an ester or amide). The lipophilic portion facilitates diffusion through membranes and correlates with potency. The hydrophilic end reversibly binds with the sodium channel in nerve membranes resulting in conduction blockade by slowing the rate of membrane depolarization. Disruption of the intermediate hydrocarbon chain initiates metabolism of the drug. For esters this occurs rapidly in the serum via hydrolysis by plasma pseudocholinesterases. Paraaminobenzoic acid (PABA) is a major metabolic product and is responsible for the higher incidence of allergies seen with ester anesthetics. Amides are metabolized in the liver by microsomal enzymes of the cytochrome P450 (CYP) system, and the kidneys excrete the much less potent metabolic products. Prilocaine, an amide anesthetic, is not recommended for use with TA, because one of its metabolites, *ortho*-toluidine, can produce methemoglobinemia at high doses. Allergic reactions to amide anesthetics are extremely rare (18–21).

Because of its efficacy and multitude of uses, lidocaine is the most commonly used and extensively studied local anesthetic drug in the United States. A detailed discussion of lidocaine pharmacology is beyond the scope of this section, but a number of important points will be stressed.

Maximum Safe Dose of Lidocaine

The maximum safe dose of lidocaine is not known. But it is clear that it should not be viewed as an absolute number in terms of dose or dosage without taking into account the myriad factors affecting its peak plasma concentration. TA is made possible because of the interplay of multiple factors that permit slow lidocaine absorption (Fig. 1).

In another pivotal study following his earlier work, Klein more closely examined absorption pharmacokinetics of dilute solutions of lidocaine and epinephrine and reached a number of important conclusions (14,22):

1. Dilution delays absorption.
2. Slow infiltration delays absorption.
3. Liposuction removes only 10–30% of the lidocaine.
4. Peak plasma lidocaine levels occurred at 12 to 14 hours after infiltration.
5. Anesthesia persists for 18 hours postoperatively.
6. The maximum safe dose was at least 35 mg/kg.

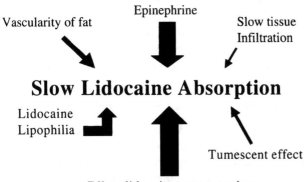

Figure 1 A number of factors contribute to permit slow lidocaine absorption, which is the key to tumescent anesthesia.

Table 2 Signs of Systemic Toxicity with Escalating Serum Concentrations of Lidocaine

Serum lidocaine (μg/mL)	Signs/symptoms of systemic toxicity
1–5	Drowsiness, lightheadedness, confusion, paresthesias, tinnitus
5–9	Vomiting, tremors, muscular fasciculations
9–12	Seizures, cardiopulmonary depression
12–20	Coma, cardiac arrest

Lipophilia

Perhaps the most important individual characteristic of lidocaine is its lipophilic nature. An IV dose of lidocaine preferentially diffuses to peripheral tissue after extensive first-pass hepatic metabolism. It follows that direct delivery to a tissue that binds it readily (i.e., adipose tissue) will lead to a more sustained effect. Couple that with a degree of dilution of the drug that further slows absorption by reducing the concentration gradient between the interstitium and intravascular compartment, and one has what can best be referred to as a "force multiplier." Klein has likened the absorption of lidocaine from the subcutaneous fat to that of a slow-release oral tablet from the gastrointestinal tract (1).

Lidocaine Toxicity

The clinical symptoms and signs of lidocaine toxicity correlate directly with its plasma concentration (Table 2). The most common initial complaint, and so the harbinger of toxicity, is drowsiness (23,24). Much of the data available on lidocaine toxicity has been garnered from studies and reports on its use in highly vascular tissue (e.g., with regional anesthetic blocks) (25) or with direct intravascular administration (e.g., when evaluating its antiarrhythmic and anticonvulsant properties). Of the limited reports available on its use specifically for induction of local cutaneous anesthesia, the evidence does point to the validity of the 7-mg/kg lidocaine with epinephrine dosage restriction, but only when used at concentrations of 1% and higher (26–30).

In a study designed to test the upper limits of maximum safe lidocaine dosage with the tumescent technique for liposuction, Ostad et al. determined that the peak plasma lidocaine concentration could be roughly estimated by the following formula (16):

Peak plasma lidocaine concentration (μg/mL) = [dose (mg)/1000] − 1.25

They concluded that a dosage of at least 55 mg/kg was safe. The study also confirmed that only a small amount of lidocaine was removed with the liposuction aspirate and that peak lidocaine concentrations occurred 4 to 8 hours postinfusion. The quicker time to peak concentrations compared with Klein's study was felt to be due to more rapid administration of the solution. Another study confirmed that slower rates of tumescent anesthetic infiltration corresponded to lower peak plasma lidocaine levels (31).

Tumescent Effect on Tissue

Hydraulic compression of lymphatics and blood vessels is also felt to play a role in limiting lidocaine absorption, but this is not an easily quantified independent parameter. A recent study seems to refute the impact of the hydraulic tissue effect, as it was determined that pressures in the subcutaneous compartment quickly dissipated after cessation of injection of the tumescent anesthetic solution, even when liposuction was not performed. The study was limited by small sample size (20 patients) and lower volumes injected (less than 250 mL to each lateral thigh of female patients) (32).

Patient Factors

Certain patient factors have a significant impact on lidocaine dose limits. The maximum safe dose for males is likely less than for females because of lower percent body fat for the former. Likewise, obese patients tolerate higher doses than do thin patients. Younger patients are able to tolerate higher doses because of better cardiovascular and hepatic function.

Lidocaine Metabolism and Drug Interactions

Of course, delayed absorption is not the whole story. Rapid and effective lidocaine metabolism is a critical component to the safe delivery of TA. As mentioned, the amide anesthetic lidocaine is metabolized by the hepatic CYP family of enzymes, specifically the isoenzymes CYP3A4 and CYP1A2. A detailed medication history to rule out concomitant use of a known CYP3A or CYP1A inhibitor (which would result in decreased lidocaine clearance and increased blood level) is of paramount importance prior to the delivery of anesthesia. General drug classes of CYP3A inhibitors include the triazole antifungals, benzodiazapines, calcium channel blockers, macrolide antibiotics, protease inhibitors, and selective serotonine reuptake inhibitors (SSRIs) (Table 3) (1,33).

   Caution is strongly advised when combining systemic anesthesia with TA. Three of the most commonly employed agents in sedation analgesia (conscious sedation) are midazolam (Versed, a benzodiazepine), fentanyl (Sublimaze, a narcotic analgesic), and propofol (Diprivan, an induction agent for general anesthesia). Both midazolam and fentanyl are metabolized via CYP3A4, and lidocaine has been shown to enhance the hypnotic effect of propofol (34–36). Other general anesthetic agents have been shown to cause elevations in plasma lidocaine levels (37).

Epinephrine

Epinephrine, also known as adrenaline, is a natural catecholamine formed in the adrenal medulla. It is a sympathomimetic agent with a potent α- and β-adrenergic agonist activity. The beneficial hemostatic effect is the direct result of peripheral vasoconstriction caused by the stimulation of α-receptors on blood vessels. β1

Table 3 Cytochrome P450 (CYP) 3A and 1A Inhibitors

CYP1A inhibitor	CYP3A inhibitor		Inhibits both
Caffeine	Alprazolam	Miconazole	Anastrozole
Ciprofloxacin	Amiodarone	Midazolam	Cimetidine
Enoxacin	Cannabidiol	Nefazodone	Clarithromycin
Mexiletine	Cyclosporine	Nelfinavir	Diltiazem
Nalidixic acid	Danazol	Nevirapine	Erythromycin
Norfloxacin	Diazepam	Nifedipine	Fluoxetine
Tacrine	Ethinyl estradiol	Norfluoxetine	Fluvoxamine
–	Felodipine	Progesterone	Grapefruit juice
–	Fluconazole	Propoxyphene	Isoniazid
–	Flurazepam	Quinidine	Ketoconazol
–	Gestodene	Saquinavir	Norfloxacin
–	Indinavir	Terfenadine	Omeprazole
–	Interferon gamma	Triazolam	Paroxetine
–	Itraconazole	Troleandomycin	Ritonavir
–	Lovastatin	Verapamil	Zileuton

Receptor stimulation on cardiac tissue leads to increased heart rate (chronotropic effect) and contractility (inotropic effect). Interestingly, at low epinephrine concentrations, stimulation of β2 receptors causes dilation of skeletal muscle arteries and increased blood flow. Epinephrine also exerts its influence on other organs and systems such as the lung, gastrointestinal tract, urinary bladder, and eye (17).

Epinephrine is best viewed as an equal partner to lidocaine with respect to its contribution to the tumescent anesthetic effect. Unlike cocaine, lidocaine and most other synthetic local anesthetic agents cause slight vasodilatation by relaxing vascular smooth muscle (possibly because of to calcium channel blockade). As expected, this leads to increased systemic absorption and accounts for its diminished duration of activity and lower dosage safety profile when used without epinephrine. The addition of epinephrine to local anesthetic solutions causes profound reduction in cutaneous blood flow via constriction of small arterioles and precapillary sphincters. This essentially eliminates clinically significant intraoperative blood loss and greatly reduces the incidence of postoperative bleeding complications. Lidocaine absorption is diminished, allowing greater doses of the drug and prolonging the postoperative anesthetic effect. The importance of epinephrine to the success and widespread clinical application of TA cannot be overemphasized.

Minimum Effective Concentration of Epinephrine

When arriving at what concentration of epinephrine should be used, it is best to think in terms of minimum effective concentration as opposed to maximum safe dose. The optimal dose is debatable and varies with the clinical situation, but for dermatologic surgery, concentrations greater than 1:200,000 are typically not necessary (38). Epinephrine is commercially available at concentrations of

1:100,000 and 1:200,000 premixed with lidocaine. Clinically, there is little difference in vasoconstriction between 1:100,000 and 1:200,000 solutions, and at concentrations greater than 1:100,000 an increase in side effects is seen (24). In contrast to an earlier study that seemed to suggest that an epinephrine dilution of 1:400,000 was no better than plain solutions of lidocaine (26), a much more recent investigation showed that concentrations as low as 1:1,000,000 resulted in a profound and statistically significant delay on the time course for lidocaine absorption (32). None of the patients underwent liposuction or any other procedure after administration of the tumescent solution. The authors concluded that the dilute concentration of lidocaine (0.1%) was the critical factor explaining the difference seen in the earlier study, where the average lidocaine concentration was 2%.

Optimal vasoconstriction with epinephrine is not achieved until at least 15 minutes after administration, and so clinically significant amounts of both lidocaine and epinephrine can be absorbed, resulting in unwanted systemic effects. It is possible that lower concentrations of lidocaine result in less vasodilatation. This underscores the importance for using the lowest effective dose for both drugs and reducing the rate of infiltration. Through careful clinical observation, Klein has arrived at an optimal epinephrine dilution of 1:2,000,000 to 1:1,000,000 (0.5–1.0 mg/L) for tumescent anesthetic solutions used for liposuction. At this concentration, a consistently excellent, prolonged vasoconstriction is achieved with a very low incidence of tachycardia, which is usually the first sign of clinically significant systemic absorption (1).

When epinephrine is used for cutaneous surgery, adverse reactions attributed solely to it are very rare. Most of those reported deal with the use of epinephrine in highly vascular areas with or without the concomitant administration of a drug that potentiates its effects. An example is blepharoplasty surgery on a patient taking the nonselective β-receptor antagonist propranolol (1,39). Both lidocaine and epinephrine diffuse rapidly through mucosal surfaces. This permits their administration via the endotracheal route during resuscitation of a patient in cardiopulmonary arrest when intravascular access is not available. As such, it is not uncommon for patients to report an "allergy" to epinephrine after a trip to the dentist, when direct injection of commercially available preparations into the highly vascular oral mucosa leads to the physiologic, albeit unpleasant, sensations of tachycardia, tremor, and anxiety. Despite the low risk of untoward events, a detailed medical history to rule out significant cardiac disease and review of the patient's medications and allergies is always indicated.

Sodium Bicarbonate

The pH of plain lidocaine is 5.0 to 7.0. Epinephrine slowly degrades in an alkaline pH, and so acidic preservatives are added to commercially available formulations of lidocaine with epinephrine, lowering the pH to approximately 4.5 (range, 3.3–5.5). This causes significantly more pain upon injection. The addition of sodium bicarbonate ($NaHCO_3$) to adjust the pH to a more physiologic range has been shown to significantly reduce the pain on infiltration of local anesthetic solutions (40,41).

The addition of NaHCO$_3$ has other benefits. At higher pH, lidocaine molecules more readily diffuse across a cell's bilayer lipid membrane. This results in quicker onset of anesthesia (42). Also, there is evidence to suggest that buffered lidocaine has enhanced antibacterial properties (43).

Normal Saline

The biggest component in terms of volume and hence the part responsible for the hydraulic tissue effect is the anesthetic solvent. The most commonly used, and preferred, solvent for TA is 0.9% sodium chloride (NaCl), also known as normal saline (NS). NS is an isotonic solution with a "physiologic" pH containing 154 mEq/L of sodium and 154 mEq/L of chloride. Lactated Ringer's (LR), which is considered by some to be more physiologic than NS, is the next most common solution used (Table 4). Because of the crystalline structure of NaCl, these fluids are also termed *crystalloids*. The choice of whether to use NS or LR comes down to personal preference and does not affect the outcome in an otherwise healthy adult undergoing conservative liposuction where less than 5 L of tumescent solution is instilled. Fluid preferences are primarily dogmatic and a product of either internal medicine or general surgery training, but they may be relevant in select cases. In the trauma patient, using a large volume of NS may aggravate a preexisting acidosis by inducing a hyperchloremic state, especially if renal function is impaired. NS is better in the setting of significant electrolyte disturbance (hyponatremia and hypochloremia) and metabolic alkalosis (44,45).

It must be remembered that crystalloid is a drug as well. Especially in the setting of TA, it wields powerful pharmacologic effects. Dynamically, the sheer volume of solution (often over a liter) required to adequately tumesce the skin raises the tissue hydrostatic pressure and contributes to the local anesthesia to a small degree by compression of peripheral cutaneous nerves. In the same manner, because of vascular compression independent of epinephrine, there is an additional anesthetic contribution by delaying lidocaine absorption. As Klein has emphasized, the subcutaneous administration of a large volume of electrolyte solution essentially eliminates the need for supplementary IV fluids in conservative

Table 4 Comparison of Electrolyte Composition (mEq/L) of Parenteral Fluids to Extracellular Fluid

Fluid	Cations				Anions		Osmolality (mOsm/L)
	Na$^+$	K$^+$	Ca^{2+}	Mg^{2+}	Cl$^-$	HCO$_3^-$	
Extracellular fluid	142	4	5	3	103	27	280–310
Normal saline	154	–	–	–	154	–	308
Lactated Ringer's	130	4	3	–	109	28	273

liposuction surgery (1,44). An appropriately administered subcutaneous tumescent dose of fluid is slowly absorbed intravascularly and then redistributed throughout the body, including the pulmonary interstitium. IV fluids are rapidly absorbed and redistributed. Fluid overload leading to pulmonary edema from careless administration of IV fluids must be guarded against. The coadministration of IV fluids when employing TA should never be considered routine.

SOLUTION PREPARATION

There is no standard or "official" recipe for the tumescent anesthetic solution. Rather, the concentrations of the various components can be varied as the clinical situation dictates, as long as one remains within the currently accepted safe limits. The balance between the minimum effective concentration of lidocaine and its maximum safe dose is sometimes delicate. To reduce the potential for toxicity, the lowest possible dose of drug "X" to achieve a desired result "Y" should be used. With respect to TA, most dermatologic surgeries can be performed at lidocaine concentrations of 0.05–0.15% (500–1500 mg/L) with epinephrine 1:1,000,000 (1 mg/L) and with no more than 5 L of anesthetic solution administered (to avoid fluid overload).

Lidocaine

Lidocaine is commercially available in concentrations ranging from 0.5% to 2%, with or without epinephrine (1:100,000 or 1:200,000), with or without methylparaben, at volumes ranging from 2 to 50 mL (10). Methylparaben is an added antiseptic preservative possibly responsible for the small number of true allergic reactions to amide anesthetics. If there is any question, then the methylparaben free (MPF) formulation should be used or the patient should be sent for allergy testing.

The concentration of lidocaine in commercially available preparations is specified in terms of gram percentage (1 g of lidocaine per 100 mL of solution). Therefore,

1% = 1 g/100 mL = 1000 mg/100 mL = 10 mg/mL

0.1% = 0.1 g/100 mL = 100 mg/100 mL = 1 mg/mL (or 1000 mg in 1 L)

Epinephrine

In commercially available preparations, epinephrine is specified in terms of grams per milliliter, so that a solution of 1:100,000 indicates 1 g of epinephrine per 100,000 mL. Therefore,

1:100,000 = 1 g/100,000 mL = 1000 mg/100,000 mL = 1 mg/100 mL

1:1000 = 1 g/1000 mL = 1000 mg/1000 mL = 1 mg/1 mL

Epinephrine for injection comes in 1:1000 ampules or premixed with lidocaine, as mentioned. To decrease the acidity of the solution and therefore the pain upon infiltration, epinephrine should be added fresh to plain lidocaine. The pH of plain lidocaine is approximately 6.4, as opposed to 4.5 for commercial lidocaine with epinephrine.

Sodium Bicarbonate

There are a variety of different commercially available preparations, all of which come without preservatives added and intended for single-dose injection (46). For ease of administration, the preferred concentration is the 8.4% solution, which is equivalent to 1 mEq/mL. A standard tumescent anesthetic formulation contains 10 mEq/mL or 10 mL of an 8.4% solution. Alkalinization causes spontaneous degradation of epinephrine, reducing the shelf life of the solution; therefore, the mixture should be prepared on the day of the procedure and not stored for later use. Also, too much alkalinization can lead to precipitation of the anesthetic, rendering it unsafe for use (may lead to tissue necrosis). If the solution appears cloudy after the addition of all the ingredients, it should be discarded.

Other Additives

The addition of other medications is a frequent, although not recommended, practice. Some add hyaluronidase to speed up the spread of the anesthetic solution through the tissue. This may in fact reduce the duration of anesthesia (47). Triamcinolone at one time was commonly added to prevent the development of "postliposuction panniculitis," a condition marked by the development of erythematous, warm and tender, sterile cutaneous nodules. Klein later determined that allowing the multiple small incision sites to heal by second intention (rather than suturing them closed) promoted better drainage of the tumescent solution and all but eliminated the problem (1,44). Because of its longer duration of anesthesia, bupivicaine is sometimes added with lidocaine. Bupivicaine is a larger, much more lipid-soluble (and therefore much less water-soluble) molecule than lidocaine. It precipitates readily after the addition of $NaHCO_3$ (48). Also, bupivicaine has been shown to have a greater potential to induce serious reentrant tachyarrhythmias that may be refractory to treatment because of prolonged binding of the molecule to the Na^+ channel (49).

Tables 5 and 6 show two standard recipes for making a 0.1% lidocaine solution containing 1 mg of epinephrine. The volumes of each ingredient can be easily adjusted to fit the clinical situation. NS is commercially available in 250-, 500-, and 1000-mL bags. The procedure planned dictates the volume used. Performing liposuction on areas of the body that are especially fibrous, such as the upper abdomen, back, and breasts, is associated with more pain and bleeding

Table 5 Recipe "A" for Tumescent Anesthetic Solution (0.1% Lidocaine with 1:1,000,000 Epinephrine)

Ingredient	Stock	Amount (mL)	Dose
Normal saline	1 L bag	889	–
1% Plain lidocaine	50 mL bottle × 2	100	1000 mg
Epinephrine 1:1000	1 ampule (1 mg/mL)	1	1 mg
8.4% Sodium bicarbonate (1 mEq/mL)	10 mL or 50 mL bottle	10	10 mEq

There is 1 mg of lidocaine for every 1 mL of solution, so the total dose of lidocaine can be easily calculated after administration of anesthetic solution.

Table 6 Recipe "B" for Tumescent Anesthetic Solution (0.1% Lidocaine with 1:1,000,000 Epinephrine)

Ingredient	Stock	Amount (mL)	Dose
Normal saline	1 L bag	890	–
1% Lidocaine with	20 mL bottle × 5	100	1000 mg
Epinephrine 1:100,000	–	–	1 mg
8.4% Sodium bicarbonate (1 mEq/mL)	10 mL or 50 mL bottle	10	10 mEq

and so often requires higher concentrations of both lidocaine and epinephrine. With respect to using TA for excisional surgery such as Mohs' micrographic surgery (MMS), one may have to wait for 30 minutes for optimal anesthetic and vasoconstrictive effect, and reinforce "hot spots" with commercially available concentrations. The volumes used for MMS are much less than that for liposuction.

The use of TA in the more highly vascular head and neck areas may potentially lead to higher plasma lidocaine levels due to quicker systemic absorption. Also, this area is more pain sensitive, so an adjustment in the standard TA recipe is indicated (Table 7). This is a useful recipe for laser cases and MMS cases with follow-on reconstruction. The total volume used rarely exceeds 200 mL.

For the standard solutions, recipe "A" is preferred primarily because its pH is closer to physiologic range. As discussed, commercial preparations of lidocaine with epinephrine are acidic solutions. The amount of $NaHCO_3$ required to bring recipe "B" into the physiologic range may cause precipitation of the lidocaine. Coleman et al. made an important point regarding volumes and expected concentrations of tumescent solutions. They showed that lidocaine concentrations may be reduced by as much as 10–14% because of the presence of extra fluid in stock formulations of both IV bags and bottles of anesthetic (50).

Table 7 Recipe for Tumescent Anesthesia of the Face (0.2% Lidocaine with 1:250,000 Epinephrine)

Ingredient	Stock	Amount (mL)	Dose
Normal saline	250 mL bag	200	–
1% Plain lidocaine	50 mL bottle	50	500 mg
Epinephrine 1:1000	1 ampule (1 mg/mL)	1	1 mg
8.4% Sodium bicarbonate (1 mEq/mL)	10 mL bottle	5	5 mEq

Two milligrams of lidocaine for every 1 mL of solution.

Standard Operating Procedure for TA

Problems with TA are rare. When they occur, they can often be linked to human error (1). As its popularity and clinical utility continues to expand, the use of TA may become as routine as any other form of local anesthesia. As the margin for error is much smaller with TA, the importance of having in place a standard operating procedure (SOP) for its use should be self-evident. There are many pitfalls waiting for the inexperienced or careless surgeon. The surgeon must consider a number of factors when planning the use of TA and have in place a clear, consistent protocol in order to ensure its safe administration.

Only the surgeon or an experienced staff member under the surgeon's direct guidance should make up the solution. All components must be checked carefully for the correct concentration prior to adding them to the solvent. We recommend stocking only 1% lidocaine so as to avert a potential overdose if 2% lidocaine is accidentally used. The solution should be made up as close as possible to the time of the planned procedure. It should not be stored for later, because epinephrine will degrade at higher pH, as mentioned previously. The solution should always be labeled appropriately, listing the doses of the additives. In case there is ever any question as to what the patient has received, all bottles, ampules, etc., of anything added to the solvent bag(s) should be saved until the end of the procedure, when the patient is appropriately recovered. The maximum safe dosage of lidocaine is predicted ahead of time, taking into account patient factors (age, sex, weight, estimate of % body fat, medical comorbidities, medications). After the procedure, document the total dose (specified in milligrams) of lidocaine and epinephrine given.

Klein currently recommends 50 mg/kg as the upper dosage limit when performing liposuction totally under local anesthesia (1). For a 60-kg woman of relatively thin build undergoing liposuction, this would dictate a maximum total lidocaine dose of 3000 mg, or 3 L of a 0.1% solution. It has been discussed that only a small percentage of the administered lidocaine is removed with the liposuction aspirate; nevertheless, if liposuction is not performed, 35 mg/kg is the currently proposed upper dosage limit (Table 8). This is an area under investigation, and so the recommendation may change (51).

Table 8 Klein's currently recommended maximum lidocaine dosage for tumescent anesthesia [less than 0.15% lidocaine with dilute (1:1,000,000) epinephrine] in a healthy adult on no interfering medications

Maximum lidocaine dosage	
With liposuction	Without liposuction
50 mg/kg	35 mg/kg

Treatment of Lidocaine Overdose

Treatment of lidocaine overdose is supportive. There is no antidote. If the patient exhibits signs and has symptoms of lidocaine toxicity, he or she should be immediately admitted to the hospital intensive care unit or telemetry unit and monitored closely for the development of cardiac dysrhythmia or onset of seizure activity for a minimum of 12 to 14 hours after the cessation of TA infiltration. It is imperative that serum lidocaine levels be followed every few hours until after the peak concentration has occurred. Seizure prophylaxis should not be instituted as antiseizure medications may interfere with lidocaine metabolism.

INSTRUMENTATION AND INFILTRATION TECHNIQUE

Advances in equipment and refinement in delivery have led to a more efficient and safe administration of the anesthetic solution since Klein's initial description of the tumescent technique. A variety of devices are available for effectively infusing the solution into the subcutaneous tissue, ranging from the simple and inexpensive to the relatively expensive and slightly more complicated.

Cannulas

The ideal cannula for infiltration has a short bevel designed to puncture the skin easily, while carrying a reduced risk of lacerating deeper tissue compared with a long-bevel instrument, such as a hypodermic needle. Spinal needles are well suited to the task of infiltration given their length and short-bevel design. A variety of gauges are available, with the 18-, 20-, and 25-gauge needles most commonly employed. The larger the diameter (12 or 14 guage) and the more blunt the tip on the infiltrating cannula, the greater the discomfort. Blunt-tipped cannulas require another instrument (such as an 11 blade) to puncture the skin and do not move through tissue as easily as their beveled counterparts. Multiport, "sprinkler"-type cannulas allow for rapid infiltration. A 15-gauge multiport needle will enable flow rates of up to 200 mL or more per minute (52).

Infiltration Assists

The simplest and least expensive infusion device is the syringe, and 10-, 20-, and 60-mL syringes for manual injection are still employed in smaller volume cases.

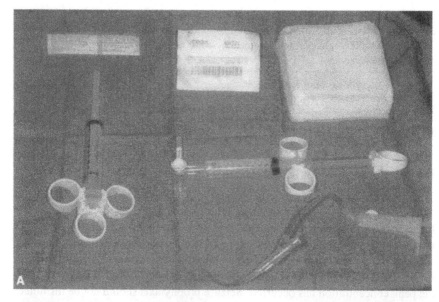

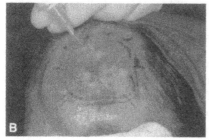
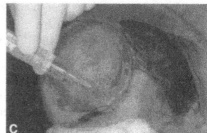

Figure 2 (**A**) A multivalve stopcock attached to a syringe is a useful device. One operator can quickly and easily refill the syringe by adjusting the valve and pulling back on the plunger. The set up is compact and can remain on the surgical tray throughout the procedure. (**B**) The tumescent effect of the solution. (**C**) Over 150 mL of a 0.1% solution was used over the course of a Mohs' procedure that lasted several hours. *Source*: Photos courtesy of Dr. Thomas Stasko.

For MMS and reconstructive surgery cases, we use a 10-mL syringe with a multiport stopcock attached to the IV bag via standard plastic infusion tubing (Fig. 2A). This allows rapid refilling of the syringe by adjusting the valve on the stopcock and can be performed by a single operator. The instrumentation can easily remain on the surgical tray, allowing for additional infiltration between stages and over the course of what may be many hours (Fig. 2B, C).

Another device, the IV power infuser, is essentially a modified sphygmomanometer. This inexpensive device fits over the IV bag and is manually inflated with a bulb pump to generate the necessary pressure to push the solution. An on/off valve is also required to control the rate of flow.

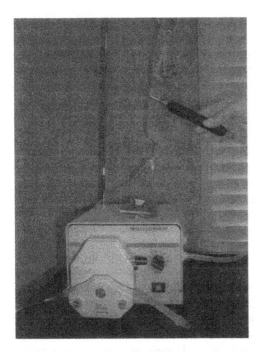

Figure 3 Variable-speed mechanical pump with multiport infiltration cannula.

A different technique for TA delivery, termed slow infusion tumescent anesthesia (SITA), was described by a group in Germany as a means for slow, precise, automated infusion (53). They used an infusomat, which is a common device found on any hospital ward and used primarily for high-volume, controlled-speed IV infusion. After positioning the needle in the center of the area to be infiltrated and setting the volume limit, the physician would often leave the room, returning from time to time to perhaps reposition the needle. Over 500 patients undergoing a variety of procedures [including sentinel node dissections ($n = 27$) and complete axillary ($n = 12$) and inguinal ($n = 17$) lymph node dissections] received this mode of delivery with a high degree of efficacy (99% experienced little or no pain) and satisfaction (97% would use it again as their sole means of anesthesia). This method was not used for liposuction anesthesia due to the longer waiting periods required for infusing larger volumes.

By far the quickest way to deliver the tumescent solution is with the use of the variable-speed peristaltic pump. This device has made the work of injecting much more efficient and less labor intensive. The Klein Infiltration System (Wells-Johnson Company, Tucson, AZ) is one such device. One person can operate these machines with the use of a pedal, keeping both hands free to facilitate the precise guidance of the cannula through the tissue. Some pumps have two pedals, which allow two operators to work at once on either side of the patient or at least prevent having to move the pedal from one side to the other when one operator is at work. Flow rates of over 500 mL/min can be easily achieved (Fig. 3).

Rate of Infiltration

The rate of TA administration should always be titrated to patient comfort. In general, patients experience more pain the more rapid the infiltration of anesthetic solution and may require additional forms of anesthesia, usually in the form of premedication with oral or intramuscular (IM) anxiolytic agents, with or without IM meperidine (Demerol) (54). Rates as high as 550 mL/min can be routinely achieved without the need for IV or general anesthesia. One must keep in mind that rapid infiltration may lead to higher peak lidocaine concentrations, although this is debatable with the use of dilute anesthetic formulations. It may only be relevant at lidocaine concentrations of 1% and higher. Of course, infiltration can be accomplished rapidly under general or IV sedation to maximize patient comfort, but with proper technique this is almost never necessary, except with the very anxious patient or one with a very low pain threshold.

Points on Technique

As one would expect, certain regions of the body are much more sensitive to infiltration than others. These are primarily the more fibrous sites such as the periumbilical and costal areas. Reducing the rate of infiltration, advancing the cannula slowly and smoothly, using smaller diameter cannulas, and increasing the concentration of anesthetic solution are techniques to keep in mind when working in more sensitive areas. Warming of the tumescent solution (in a microwave oven or hot water bath) prior to infusion has been shown to significantly improve the pain associated with infiltration compared with that of a room temperature solution (55,56). This also prevents the core body temperature from lowering as can occur if even room temperature solutions are used. Chilled solutions should never be used. Care must also be taken not to overheat the solution.

Precise, uniform infiltration of the anesthetic into the subcutaneous fat is critical to the safe and effective use of TA. It should be infiltrated in a radiating pattern from a central point, pushing fluid as the cannula is advanced. As many entry points as are necessary can be made as these sites almost always heal without a noticeable scar. The infiltration should begin in the deepest planes of fatty tissue to facilitate better diffusion of the solution once instilled. Also, starting too superficial interferes with an appreciation of the fat/muscle interface and may lead to inadvertent injury.

The optimum volume of anesthetic to use and the time over which to infiltrate it are a direct function of what will provide complete, local anesthesia. It differs from region to region, patient to patient, and procedure to procedure. Remember to calculate the maximum safe dose for each patient prior to starting the infiltration, and always be aware of when that dose (volume) is nearing.

CLINICAL APPLICATIONS

The benefits inherent in the TAT, namely, safe delivery of local anesthesia to a large region, profound reduction in operative bleeding, prolonged postoperative anesthesia, and the hydraulic changes to the target tissue have led to an explosion of its use outside of liposuction surgery (Table 9). It may be used as the only form of anesthesia or may be employed in addition to regional nerve blockade, sedation analgesia, or general anesthesia. Many factors (e.g., patient pain threshold and anxiety level, body area treated, specific procedure performed, and technique and temperament of the surgeon) have an impact on what type and degree of anesthesia will be used for any given procedure. But patient safety is paramount. If potentially harmful medications can be avoided, they should be.

Without question, TA is used most frequently in conjunction with liposuction surgery. Klein and others strongly emphasize that when the tumescent technique for liposuction is employed in the proper manner, complete anesthesia can be achieved entirely with the tumescent solution in the vast majority of patients, obviating the need for systemic anesthesia. Unfortunately, many procedures amenable to local anesthesia are still performed under systemic anesthesia. The risk of general anesthesia is well documented, although it is often difficult to determine the exact cause of the deaths reported. In American Society of Anesthesiologists (ASA) class I patients (healthy, no disease), the risk of death due to systemic anesthesia is estimated at one in 10,000 to 20,000 (1,57–59). There have been no reported deaths linked solely to the administration of TA, whether performed for liposuction or some other procedure (1,60,61).

With or without systemic anesthesia, the use of TA is now considered the standard of care for liposuction. But outside its use for liposuction, it is difficult to gauge just how consistently and effectively TA is used in day-to-day practice, and whether its use will supplant systemic anesthesia for other procedures. Over a one-year period, a group of dermatologic surgeons from Israel reported using it in a total of 242 cases ranging from large reconstructive surgeries ($n = 75$) to a variety of cosmetic procedures, including laser resurfacing ($n = 50$), liposuction ($n = 40$), hair transplantation ($n = 30$), blepharoplasties ($n = 20$), face lifts ($n = 10$), as well as mini-abdominoplasty ($n = 7$) and breast augmentation ($n = 5$), among a few others (62). In 90% of the cases, only TA was used, and there were no adverse events reported. Without TA, a number of those cases would almost certainly have required some form of systemic anesthesia.

Dermatologic surgeons have been at the forefront of new, innovative applications for TA. Its utility for ambulatory phlebectomy and other venous surgery has been detailed in several reports (63–66). It has been incorporated into dermabrasion (67,68), chemical peels, and laser resurfacing (69). Our own experience with TA for full-face laser resurfacing has shown it to be somewhat difficult to use as the only means of anesthesia. Most patients require nerve blocks with or without IV sedation as well. An oral and maxillofacial surgery group recently described its experience with TA for facial laser resurfacing (70). Several patients were able to tolerate the procedure entirely under local anesthesia with a modified tumescent technique, although most required IV sedation as well.

TA has proved to be especially useful for surgery on the scalp (68). With conventional local anesthesia, large areas can be difficult to anesthetize without multiple needle sticks or nerve blocks. With TA, the scalp can be completely

Table 9 Reported Uses of Tumescent Anesthesia with or Without Systemic Anesthesia

Procedure	TA	TA + SA
Abdominoplasty	X	X
Ambulatory phlebectomy	X	
Breast surgery		
Augmentation mammaplasty	X	
Implant removal and capsulectomy		X
Mastectomy		X
Reduction mammaplasty	X	X
TRAM flap breast reconstruction		X
Burn surgery		X
Cervicofacial rhytidectomy	X	X
Chemical peels	X	
Dermabrasion	X	
Hair transplantation	X	
Laser resurfacing	X	X
Liposuction		
Cosmetic and noncosmetic applications	X	X
Lymph node dissection	X	
Mohs' micrographic surgery	X	
Pressure ulcer closure		X
Reconstructive surgery (flaps and grafts) after skin cancer removal	X	
Rhinophymectomy	X	
Scalp surgery	X	
Sentinel lymph node biopsy	X	
Split thickness skin graft harvesting	X	

Abbreviations: TA, tumescent anesthesia; SA, systemic anesthesia.

anesthetized with only a few puncture sites. Given its rich vascular supply, the scalp is ideally suited for TA. Hydraulic effects (elevation, magnification, compression) on the tissue in this area go a long way toward facilitating the subsequent surgical procedure. The large fluid volume causes hydrodissection of the galea aponeurotica from the pericranium and facilitates the wide undermining often required with scalp reductions or large flaps to cover defects after tumor removal. Hair transplant surgery, especially with the newer technique of micrografting, takes advantage of all that TA has to offer (71–73).

A definite indication for TA is any prolonged or extensive dermatologic surgical procedure where one may expect to exceed the dosage of 7 mg/kg of 1% lidocaine with epinephrine (74,75). TA lends itself especially well to MMS, which can extend over many hours before tumor extirpation is complete. In addition, reconstruction of the resultant defect is performed immediately after MMS in the vast majority of cases, which may add substantially to the operative

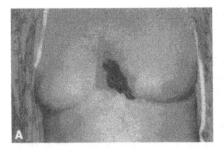 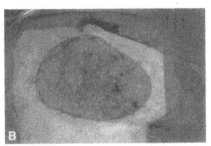

Figure 4 Before (**A**) and after (**B**) Mohs' micrographic surgery for extensive basal cell carcinoma on the chest. A total of 310 mL of tumescent anesthetic (0.1% lidocaine with 1:500,000 epinephrine) was used in addition to 27 mL of 1% lidocaine with 1:300,000 epinephrine. *Source*: Photos courtesy of Dr. Thomas Stasko.

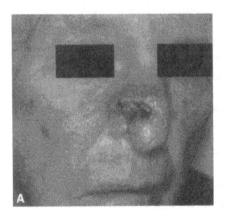 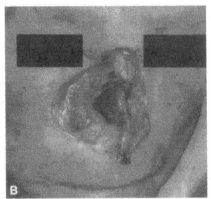

Figure 5 Before (**A**) and after (**B**) Mohs' micrographic surgery for recurrent, infiltrating basal cell carcinoma on the nose. A total of 130 mL of tumescent anesthetic (0.1% lidocaine with 1:500,000 epinephrine) was used in addition to 24 mL of 1% lidocaine with 1:300,000 epinephrine. *Source*: Photos courtesy of Dr. Thomas Stasko.

time. Figures 4 and 5 show two MMS cases in which TA was used at our institution. The chest of this particular patient was an especially ideal location given its fatty nature. Note the bloodless surgical field.

The utility of TA for reconstructive surgery has been demonstrated. In a study involving 86 patients referred for moderately complex reconstructive surgery after skin cancer removal, Acosta reported that 95% experienced the same or less pain on infiltration with TA compared to conventional local anesthesia. During surgery, 90% experienced no pain after the initial administration of anesthetic. The other 10% required additional TA without the need for any other type of anesthesia. The prolonged postoperative anesthetic effect was excellent: For 24 hours after surgery, 98% reported no or only mild pain (required no analgesics). Tissue swelling had reduced by at least 90% by the first postoperative day in every patient. As expected, intraoperative and postoperative hemostasis was excellent. There was only one reported complication: a small, localized hematoma (7). Field has described a useful technique for harvesting split thickness skin grafts with TA (76). A plastic surgery group reported on its use in helping with anesthesia and hemostasis in reconstructing a large pressure ulcer (77).

Surgery on the breast is well suited for TA given the fatty nature of this tissue. Reports of augmentation and reduction mammaplasty performed under TA and without the use of IV or inhalational anesthesia have been reported (61). The use of TA in conjunction with cosmetic facial surgery, primarily cervicofacial rhytidectomy, is becoming much more commonplace. The first report of TA for facelifts was by Brody in 1994 (78). Since then, there have been a number of reports detailing its use. The hemostatic effect and help with flap elevation from tissue hydrodissection are important benefits. Well-respected, academic plastic surgeons now consider it a critical adjunct for safe, successful facelift surgery (79).

An increase in TA use among nondermatologic surgeons seems to relate primarily to the hemostatic benefits (6,9,80,81). Less attention is paid to the anesthetic power of TA to limit or even eliminate the need for systemic anesthesia in many cases. Interestingly, even with the proven track record of safety and cost-effectiveness, the advent of TA does not seem to have affected *where* most surgeons perform their surgery, although there are a few exceptions (82). Even though the literature suggests that surgeons of all stripes are routinely using TA, nondermatologic surgeons still combine it with some form of systemic anesthesia. On the other hand, as dermatologic surgery remains a primarily outpatient, office-based specialty, a large number of procedures traditionally performed only in hospital operating rooms by plastic surgeons are now routinely and safely performed by dermatologic surgeons in an office, under local anesthesia.

SUMMARY

Jeffrey A. Klein, the originator of TA states: "The essence of the tumescent technique is the direct infiltration of very dilute (0.05–0.15%) lidocaine with epinephrine into an area of subcutaneous fat, resulting in an unprecedented slow rate of systemic lidocaine absorption." (1) Safety is perhaps the principal hallmark of TA. The safe delivery of a large dose of local anesthetic that eliminates the need for systemic anesthesia in many cases and provides a hemostatic benefit that further enhances the safety of the procedure performed by reducing surgical blood loss. There is no standard recipe for the anesthetic solution. The formulation may differ from one body site to the other, and from one procedure to the next, with the primary difference being the variation in the concentration of either/both the lidocaine or epinephrine as a means to titrate the anesthetic and vasoconstrictive effects. The usefulness of this specific form of local anesthesia has been demonstrated with numerous surgical procedures.

TA is, without a question, one of the major advances in the practice of dermatologic surgery.

REFERENCES

1. Klein JA. Tumescent Technique: Tumescent Anesthesia and Microcannular Liposuction. St. Louis: Mosby, 2000.
2. Klein JA. The tumescent technique for liposuction surgery. Am J Cosmet Surg 1987; 4:263–267.
3. Rao RB, Ely SF, Hoffman RS. Deaths related to liposuction. N Engl J Med 1999; 340:1471–1475.
4. Rigel DS, Wheeland RG. Deaths related to liposuction. N Engl J Med 1999; 341: 1001–1002.
5. Platt MS, Cohle SD, Kohler LJ. Semantic differences between "tumescent liposuction," "tumescent anesthesia," and "tumescent technique." J Forensic Sci 2003; 48:1206.
6. Paige KT, Bostwick J III, Bried JT. TRAM flap breast reconstruction: tumescent technique reduces blood loss and transfusion requirement. Plast Reconstr Surg 2004; 113:1645–1649.
7. Acosta AE. Clinical parameters of tumescent anesthesia in skin cancer reconstructive surgery: a review of 86 patients. Arch Dermatol 1997; 133:451–454.
8. Karacalar A, Karacalar S, Cepni H. Use of the real tumescent technique: anesthesia in the surgical management of lip cancer. Ann Plast Surg 2003; 50:107–108.
9. Robertson RD, Bond P, Wallace B, et al. The tumescent technique to significantly reduce blood loss during burn surgery. Burns 2001; 27:835–838.
10. Xylocaine (lidocaine HCL injection): maximum recommended dosages. In: Physicians' Desk Reference. 55th ed. Montvale, NJ: Medical Economics, 2001.
11. Klein JA. Anesthesia for liposuction in dermatologic surgery. J Dermatol Surg Oncol 1988; 14:1124–1132.
12. Gorgh T. Xylocaine—A new local anesthetic. Anaesthesia 1949; 4:4–9.
13. Lillis PJ. Liposuction surgery under local anesthesia: limited blood loss and minimal lidocaine absorption. J Dermatol Surg Oncol 1988; 14:1145–1148.
14. Klein JA. Tumescent technique for regional anesthesia permits lidocaine doses of 35 mg/kg for liposuction. J Dermatol Surg Oncol 1990; 16:248–263.
15. Samdal F, Amland PF, Bugge JF. Plasma lidocaine levels during suction-assisted lipectomy using large doses of dilute lidocaine with epinephrine. Plast Reconstr Surg 1994; 93:1217–1223.
16. Ostad A, Kageyama N, Moy R. Tumescent anesthesia with a lidocaine dose of 55 mg/kg is safe for liposuction. Dermatol Surg 1996; 22:921–927.
17. Hardman JG, Limbird LE, eds. Goodman & Gilman: The Pharmacological Basis of Therapeutics. 10th ed. New York: McGraw-Hill, 2001.
18. McCarthy RJ, Tuman KJ. Local anesthetics. In: White PF, ed. Textbook of Intravenous Anesthesia. Baltimore: Williams & Wilkins, 1997:259–278.
19. Butterworth JF, Strichartz GR. Molecular mechanism of local anesthesia: a review. Anesthesiology 1990; 72:711–734.
20. Covino BG. Pharmacology of local anesthetic agents. Br J Anaesth 1986; 58:701–716.
21. Grekin RC, Auletta MJ. Local anesthesia in dermatologic surgery. J Am Acad Dermatol 1988; 19:599–614.

22. Klein JA. Tumescent technique for local anesthesia improves safety in large-volume liposuction. Plast Reconstr Surg 1993; 92:1085–1098.
23. Lie KI, Wellers HJ, van Capelle FJ, et al. Lidocaine in the prevention of primary ventricular fibrillation: a double blind, randomized study of 212 consecutive patients. N Engl J Med 1974; 291:1324–1326.
24. de Jong RH. Local Anesthetics. 2nd ed. Springfield, IL: Charles C. Thomas, 1977.
25. Grimes DA, Cates WJr. Deaths from paracervical anesthesia for first trimester abortion, 1972–1975. N Engl J Med 1976; 295:1397–1399.
26. Scott DB, Jebson PJR, Braid DP, et al. Factors affecting plasma levels of lignocaine and prilocaine. Br J Anaesth 1972; 44:1040–1049.
27. Piveral K. Systemic lidocaine absorption during liposuction. Plast Reconstr Surg 1987; 80:643.
28. Nattel S, Rinkenberger RL, Lehrman LL, et al. Therapeutic blood lidocaine concentrations after local anesthesia for cardiac electrophysiologic studies. N Engl J Med 1979; 301:418–420.
29. Bashien G. Use of excessive lidocaine concentrations for local anesthesia. N Engl J Med 1980; 302:122.
30. Kosowsky BE, Mufti S, Grewal GS. Effect of local lidocaine anesthesia on ventricular escape intervals during permanent pacemaker implantation in patients with complete heart block. Am J Cardiol 1983; 51:101–104.
31. Butterwick KJ, Goldman MP, Sriprachya-Anunt S. Lidocaine levels during the first two hours of infiltration of dilute anesthetic solution for tumescent liposuction: rapid versus slow delivery. Dermatol Surg 1999; 25:681–685.
32. Rubin JP, Bierman C, Rosow CE, et al. The tumescent technique: the effect of high tissue pressure and dilute epinephrine on absorption of lidocaine. Plast Reconstr Surg 1999; 103:990–996.
33. Katz HI. Dermatologist's Guide to Adverse Therapeutic Interactions. Revised ed. Philadelphia: Lippincott-Raven, 1997.
34. Wandel C, Bocker R, Bohrer H. Midazolam is metabolized by at least three different cytochrome P450 enzymes. Br J Anesth 1994; 73:658–661.
35. Bartkowski RR, McDonell TE. Prolonged alfentanil effect following erythromycin administration. Anesthesiology 1990; 73:566–568.
36. Ben Shlomo I, Tverskoy G, Cherniavsky G. Hypnotic effect of i.v. propofol is enhanced by i.m. administration of either lignocaine or bupivicaine. Br J Anaesth 1997; 78:375–377.
37. Bentley JB, Glass S, Gandolfi AJ. The influence of halothane on lidocaine pharmacokinetics in man. Anesthesiology 1983; 59:246.
38. Siegel RJ, Vistnes LM, Iverson RE. Effective hemostasis with less epinephrine: an experimental and clinical study. Plast Reconstr Surg 1973; 51:129–133.
39. Foster CA, Aston SJ. Propranolol-epinephrine interaction: a potential disaster. Plast Reconstr Surg 1983; 72:74–78.
40. McKay W, Morris R, Mushlin P. Sodium bicarbonate attenuates pain on skin infiltration with lidocaine, with or without epinephrine. Anesth Analg 1987; 66:572–574.
41. Stewart JH, Cole GW, Klein JA. Neutralized lidocaine with epinephrine for local anesthesia. J Dermatol Surg Oncol 1989; 15:1081–1083.
42. DiFazio CA, Carron H, Grosslight KR, et al. Comparison of pH-adjusted lidocaine solutions for epidural anesthesia. Anesth Analg 1986; 65:760–764.

43. Thompson KD, Welykyj S, Massa MC. Antibacterial activity of lidocaine in combination with a bicarbonate buffer. J Dermatol Surg Oncol 1993; 19:216–220.
44. Klein JA. Anesthetic formulation of tumescent solutions. Dermatol Clin 1999; 17:751–759.
45. Cohen RD, Simpson R. Lactate metabolism. Anesthesiology 1975; 43:661–673.
46. Package insert. Sodium bicarbonate injection, USP. Abbott Laboratories, Chicago, IL 60064.
47. Narins RS. Liposuction and anesthesia. Dermatol Clin 1990; 8:421–424.
48. Robinson J, Fernando R. Chemical stability of bupivicaine, lidocaine, and epinephrine in pH-adjusted solutions. Anesthesia 2000; 55:853–858.
49. Moller RA, Covino BG. Cardiac electrophysiologic effects of lidocaine and bupivicaine. Anesth Analg 1988; 67:107.
50. Coleman WP IV, Flynn TC, Coleman KM. When one liter does not equal 1000 milliliters: implications for the tumescent technique. Dermatol Surg 2000; 26: 1024–1028.
51. Klein JA. Tumescent local anesthesia peak serum lidocaine concentrations without liposuction. ASDS-ACMMSCO Combined Annual Meeting. September 30–October 3, 2004; San Diego, CA.
52. Bernstein G. Instrumentation for liposuction. Dermatol Clin 1999; 17:735–749.
53. Breuninger H, Wehner-Caroli J. Slow infusion tumescent anesthesia. Dermatol Surg 1998; 24:759–763.
54. Hanke CW, Coleman WP, Lillis PJ, et al. Infusion rates and levels of premedication in tumescent liposuction. Dermatol Surg 1997; 23:1131–1134.
55. Fialkor JA, McDougal EP. Warmed local anesthetic reduces pain on infiltration. Ann Plast Surg 1996; 36:11–13.
56. Kaplan B, Moy RL. Comparison of room temperature and warmed local anesthetic solution for tumescent liposuction. A randomized, double-blind study. Dermatol Surg 1996; 22:707–709.
57. Taylor G, Larson CP, Prestwick R. Unexpected cardiac arrest during anesthesia and surgery. JAMA 1976; 235:2758–2760.
58. Keenan RL, Boyan CP. Cardiac arrest due to anesthesia: a study of incidence and causes. JAMA 1985; 253:2373–2377.
59. Warner MA, Shields SE, Chute CG. Major morbidity and mortality within one month of ambulatory surgery and anesthesia. JAMA 1993; 270:1437–1441.
60. Hanke CW, Bernstein G, Bullock S. Safety of tumescent liposuction in 15,336 patients. National survey results. Dermatol Surg 1995; 21:459–462.
61. Housman TS, Lawrence N, Mellen BG, et al. The safety of liposuction: results of a national survey. Dermatol Surg 2002; 28:971–978.
62. Namias A, Kaplan B. Tumescent anesthesia for dermatologic surgery: cosmetic and noncosmetic procedures. Dermatol Surg 1998; 24:755–758.
63. Cohn MS, Seiger E, Goldman S. Ambulatory phlebectomy using the tumescent technique for local anesthesia. Dermatol Surg 1995; 21:315–318.
64. Smith SR, Goldman MP. Tumescent anesthesia in ambulatory phlebectomy. Dermatol Surg 1998; 24:453–456.
65. Keel D, Goldman MP. Tumescent anesthesia in ambulatory phlebectomy: addition of epinephrine. Dermatol Surg 1999; 25:371–372.

66. Proebstle TM, Paepcke U, Weisel G, et al. High ligation and stripping of the long saphenous vein using the tumescent technique for local anesthesia. Dermatol Surg 1998; 24:149–153.
67. Goodman G. Dermabrasion using tumescent anesthesia. J Dermatol Surg Oncol 1994; 20:802–807.
68. Coleman WPIII, Klein JA. Use of the tumescent technique for scalp surgery, dermabrasion, and soft tissue reconstruction. J Dermatol Surg 1992; 18:130–135.
69. Field LM. Re: the long pulsed Er:YAG laser and intravenous sedation versus dermabrasion (or laser) utilizing tumescent anesthesia for colloid milium. Dermatol Surg 2002; 28:780.
70. Potter JK, Finn R, Cillo J. Modified tumescent technique for outpatient facial laser resurfacing. J Oral Maxillofac Surg 2004; 62:829–833.
71. Unger WP. What's new in hair replacement surgery. Dermatol Clin 1996; 14:783–802.
72. Hunstad JP. The tumescent technique facilitates hair micrografting. Aesthetic Plast Surg 1996; 20:43–48.
73. Field LM, Namias A. Bilevel tumescent anesthetic infiltration for hair transplantation. Dermatol Surg 1997; 23:289–290.
74. Holt P, Motley R, Field L. Tumescent technique for anesthesia in skin surgery. Br J Dermatol 1995; 133:46–48.
75. Thomas J. Adjunctive tumescent technique in massive resections. Aesthetic Plast Surg 2001; 25:343–346.
76. Field L, Hrabovsky T. Harvesting split thickness grafts with tumescent anesthesia. Dermatol Surg 1997; 23:62.
77. Han H, Few J, Fine NA. Use of the tumescent technique in pressure ulcer closure. Plast Reconstr Surg 2002; 110:711–712.
78. Brody GS. The tumescent technique for facelift. Plast Reconstr Surg 1994; 94:563.
79. LaTrenta GS, Talmor M. Tumescent cervicofacial rhytidectomy. Perspect Plast Surg 2001; 15:47–59.
80. Solomon MP. Tumescent technique as an adjunct to breast implant removal and capsulectomy. Ann Plast Surg 2000; 44:495–497.
81. Worland RG. Expanded utilization of the tumescent technique for mastectomy. Plast Reconstr Surg 1996; 98:1321.
82. Abramson DL. Tumescent abdominoplasty: an ambulatory office procedure. Aesthetic Plast Surg 1998; 22:404–407.

7

Local Anesthesia for Children

Thierry Pirotte and Francis Veyckemans

*Department of Anesthesiology, Cliniques
Universitaires Saint-Luc, Brussels, Belgium*

INTRODUCTION

The anatomic and physiologic capacities to respond to nociception develop early in fetal life and acute behavioral and biochemical responses to tissue damage are well documented in preterm and full-term neonates (1). Moreover, a child's first experience with unrelieved pain will affect how it reacts to subsequent painful events: for example, Taddio et al. noted that neonates circumcised without anesthesia show an increased behavioral response to routine vaccination at four or six months of age when compared with neonates circumcised with local anesthesia (2). Last, children often learn by associating neutral with nonneutral stimuli: a neutral event like visiting a doctor can thus easily be associated with a nonneutral stimulus such as pain, fear, and anxiety if the visit includes a painful procedure. A first bad medical experience can thus influence a child's attitude toward medicine for a long time. It is thus one of our responsibilities, as medical practitioners, to handle pediatric patients with extreme care not only for present humanitarian reasons but also because they are future adults.

The growing use of short office-based procedures to cure skin problems in children both necessitates and can partly be attributed to the advances in pediatric local anesthesia and psychologic preparation.

This chapter is divided in two parts: the first describes the basic anatomic, physiologic, and pharmacologic differences between children and adults regarding local anesthesia—the fact that infants and children are not "little adults" will be highlighted. The second part gives a practical overview of the local anesthesia and sedation techniques that can be used for pediatric dermatologic surgery in order to help the reader choosing the best agent and technique with regard to efficacy, safety, and feasibility in children.

THE PEDIATRIC PATIENT: IMPLICATIONS REGARDING LOCAL ANESTHESIA

For the basic pharmacology of local anesthetics (LA) and their additives, we send the reader back to chapters 1 and 2. The purpose of the first part of this chapter is to highlight the anatomic, physiologic, and pharmacologic implications of infancy and childhood regarding local anesthesia (Table 1).

Anatomic Considerations

The most superficial layer of the skin, the stratum corneum, is the foundation of the epidermal permeability barrier. The stratum corneum of premature neonates is

Table 1 Major Anatomic and Physiologic Features of the Pediatric Period and Their Implications Regarding Local Anesthesia

Anatomic, physiologic, and metabolic features	Clinical consequences and specific dangers	Implications for local anesthesia
Incomplete myelinization of nerve fibers	Easier penetration	Diluted solution more effective, reduced latency but shorter duration
Loose attachment of perineural sheaths	Increased spread along nerve paths with risk of distant nerve blocks	Less volumes required for peripheral nerve blocks but larger volumes for central blocks
Increased cardiac output and local blood flow	Increased systemic absorption	Reduced duration of effects, increased effectiveness of epinephrine
High distribution volume	–	Compensates partly the decreased plasma protein binding of LA
Enzyme immaturity	Slower metabolism of amides Danger of drug accumulation in case of repeated injections	Smaller reinjection doses

much thinner and less effective than in full-term infants and adults. At 34 weeks' gestational age, the barrier is deemed to be mature. In infants born at less than 34 weeks' gestational age, rapid epidermal cell differentiation occurs in the first postnatal weeks (3). Difficulties with fluid homeostasis, thermoregulation, infection control, but also systemic toxicity after percutaneous absorption have to be expected in this population. Although several studies show that topical anesthesia can, with adapted guidelines (see further), be used in preterm infants, special care should be taken with regard to their skin fragility; for example, Gourrier et al. (4) recommend using EMLA® with a nonadhesive transparent dressing instead of Tegaderm® to avoid tissue damage on removal, and Long (5) proposes a novel tetracaine patch providing a more secure and less aggressive means of skin attachment.

Nerve fiber envelopes are not fully differentiated at birth. The myelinization process begins in the cervical neuromeres during the fetal period and progressively extends downward and upward, but is not achieved until the 12th year of life. Lack of myelin favors penetration of LA, a process enhanced further by the reduced size of nerve fibers and the shorter distance between successive nodes of Ranvier. LA indeed need to block more than two or three nodes to interrupt nerve conduction in myelinated axons. Moreover, in infants, the endoneurium is loose and easily crossed by LA both from outside to inside and from inside to outside. Nerve blockade thus occurs more quickly, even with low-concentration solutions, but usually lasts for a shorter time than in older children. As the child grows, the endoneurium becomes more enriched in connective tissues, and thus less permeable. Not only the latency of LA but also the duration of their effect increases with age.

Developmental Pharmacology of LA

Most pediatric pharmacologic studies on LA have been performed on small numbers of patients undergoing either a single-shot (caudal, femoral, axillary, ilioinguinal) administration or a continuous epidural infusion of the drug studied. The application of their results to the use of LA in dermatologic surgery is thus difficult, and only the information most relevant to this special field is summarized hereafter (6).

Metabolism of Ester-Type Local Anesthetics

The ester-type LA are quickly metabolized in the blood by plasma cholinesterase (also called butyrylcholinesterase or pseudocholinesterase (PCHE)), which is mainly synthesized in the liver. Their duration of action and toxicity is thus increased in patients with inherited deficiencies of PCHE (the incidence of homozygous forms in the Caucasian subjects varies from 1/2500 to 1/150,000). The metabolism of ester LA may be delayed in neonates and infants because of their lower PCHE levels but the clinical result is of little importance. It should be noted that one of the end products of that metabolism is para-aminobenzoic acid, which can induce allergic reactions.

Metabolism of Amide-Type Local Anesthetics

The amide-type LA undergo exclusive hepatic metabolism and depend thus on both enzymatic activity and liver blood flow. They are metabolized by the cytochrome P450 system, mainly the CYP 3A4 subtype but also CYP 1A2 for ropivacaine and levobupivacaine. Although fetal CYP 3A7 is able to metabolize amide LA in the neonatal period, the CYP system is immature before the age of 3 weeks and becomes fully mature around one year; that is why the clearance of amide LA is decreased during the first six months of age.

Some of the metabolites are active and their accumulation can cause toxic effects. For example, the metabolism of lidocaine produces monoethylglycin-exylidide, which accumulates during continuous infusion of lidocaine and has proconvulsive properties. Prilocaine is metabolized in 4- and 6-hydroxytoluidine, which can lead to methemoglobinemia. Because the activity of methemoglobin reductase is low in infants less than six months (6), the use of prilocaine is not recommended below that age, except in the form of EMLA cream provided the recommendations for its use are observed (see EMLA further).

Regarding liver blood flow, the metabolism of drugs with a high hepatic extraction ratio (>60%, e.g., lidocaine with a value of 65%) depends mainly of liver blood flow and thus cardiac output. On the other hand, the metabolism of drugs with a low hepatic extraction ratio (e.g., bupivacaine with a value of 35%) depends on the free fraction present in the plasma and on the metabolic capacity of the hepatic microsomes. The greater liver mass of children two to five years old explains the increased clearance of many drugs, including LA, in that age group.

Pharmacokinetics

At its site of administration (skin, mucosa, epidural space), the concentration of the LA is very high: its local disposition contributes to its onset and duration of action but also to its systemic absorption. Differences in systemic absorption are due to binding to local tissue (e.g., tissue proteins, epidural fat that acts as a reservoir) or to vascularity (e.g., mucosae, intercostal space, use of epinephrine).

After systemic absorption into the bloodstream, a significant amount of the amide LA is trapped in the lungs (7). This buffering capacity of the lung is limited and transient and the LA is quickly released back into the circulation; that is why the arterial concentration of an amide LA is lower than its central venous concentration during the first 15 minutes after its intercostal or epidural administration. In the same way, its peripheral venous concentrations are lower than its arterial ones up to at least 30 minutes after the injection (8). The majority of pediatric pharmacologic studies on amide LA are based, for obvious practical

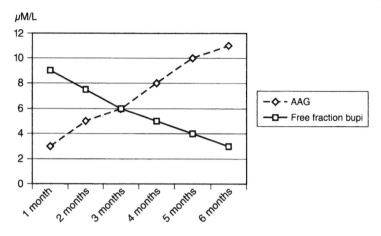

μM/L

Figure 1 Serum levels of free bupivacaine and of AAG in infants less than six months after a single dose bupivacaine by the caudal route. *Abbreviation*: AAG, α_1-acid glycoprotein. *Source*: Modified from Ref. 9.

reasons, on the measurement of peripheral venous concentrations and thus underestimate their early arterial peak concentration. The fact that the pulmonary buffering capacity is partially bypassed explains why there is an increased risk of early systemic toxicity in infants and children with an intracardiac right to left shunt.

Because neonates and infants have a greater body water content than children and adults, the volume of distribution of LA is almost twice as great in that population. This decreases the peak concentrations observed and contributes to the reduced clearance of the LA in neonates and infants.

In blood, LA bind to red blood cells and serum proteins with a binding ratio varying between 65% and 96%: the free (unbound) concentration of the LA undergoes hepatic metabolism and is able to diffuse into the brain and heart to produce systemic effects (see acute toxicity). The two main serum proteins that bind LA are albumin and α_1-acid glycoprotein (AAG or orosomucoid). Albumin has a low affinity but a high capacity for binding LA, while AAG has a high affinity but a low capacity.

In neonates and infants, blood AAG concentration is low and does not reach adult levels before 10 months of age; the free fraction of circulating LA is thus increased in that age group. For example, the free fraction of bupivacaïne is three to six times greater in neonates than in infants older than six months (9) (Fig. 1). The increased volume of distribution of LA in neonates and infants only partially compensates for the decreased protein binding. Moreover, AAG is a stress protein that is synthetized in the liver in response to stimuli such as infection or trauma, or during the postoperative period (10); the postoperative inflammatory response dramatically increases the AAG levels. This explains why, in case of continuous infusion of a LA solution in infants, a progressive increase of both total and free concentrations of the LA is observed but that its free fraction (in %) remains stable or decreases, thanks to the postoperative increase in AAG synthesis (11). For example, in case of continuous epidural infusion of bupivacaine in infants, the mean concentration of total and free bupivacaine increases from 0.53 and 0.07 µg/mL after the initial injection to 1.77 and 0.14 µg/mL, respectively, after 48 hours of infusion; the mean free fraction decreases from 13.2% to 7.9%. Almost all clinical circumstances that decrease serum albumin levels also induce an increase of AAG that compensates for hypoalbuminemia; however, great care should be observed in children with nephrotic syndrome because it leads to an important decrease in both AAG and albumin.

Although LA have a low affinity for red blood cells, their binding to them becomes important when binding to the serum proteins becomes saturated, i.e., when levels of AAG are low or when toxic blood concentrations occur. This buffer system is thus not efficient in infants less than six months, in whom both physiologic anemia and low AAG levels are present. For reasons that are still unknown, in children rectal premedication with diazepam increases the plasma concentrations measured after the caudal administration of bupivacaine (0.84 ± 0.08 µg/mL vs. 0.48 ± 0.05 µg/mL, $p = 0.005$) but not lidocaine; this interaction is not observed following rectal midazolam (12). Whether the same pharmacologic interaction occurs with different routes of administration of benzodiazepines or with levobupivacaine or ropivacaine is not known.

Adjuvant Drugs

Epinephrine.   Epinephrine is the most commonly used adjuvant. It is added to the LA solution to decrease and delay the peak blood concentration of the LA and prolong its duration of action. This effect is more important with short acting LA such as lidocaine than with bupivacaine, ropivacaine, and levobupivacaine. Many anesthesiologists also add epinephrine 1/200,000 or 1/400,000 to use a "test dose" when performing an epidural or peripheral nerve block: the electrocardiographic and systemic effects of epinephrine can provide early signs of accidental intravascular administration of the solution.

However, epinephrine should not be used when infiltrating skin in anatomic locations where arterial vascularization is terminal, such as digits and toes, the penis, the pinna of the ear, and some blocks of the face (e.g., infraorbital nerve block), because tissue necrosis can occur.

Clonidine.   Clonidine at a dose of 1 to 2 µg/kg is often added when performing an epidural or peripheral nerve block to increase the duration and quality of the block obtained. At those doses, only mild sedation is observed in children.

ACUTE TOXICITY OF LOCAL ANESTHETICS IN CHILDREN

Systemic toxicity of a LA can occur after any route of administration: subcutaneous, mucosal, plexus or nerve block, or epidural block. The clinical signs of systemic toxicity occur when a so-called toxic threshold plasma concentration is exceeded because of accidental intravascular injection or overdose (too much drug administered at the good place) (13).

The symptoms and signs of toxicity are caused by the action of the LA on the sodium channels of other excitable membranes, i.e., the brain and the heart. They vary with the blood levels of unbound LA achieved; neurologic signs usually precede cardiovascular signs, but because young children are either unable to report reliably the first symptoms of neurologic involvement or have their local block performed under sedation or general anesthesia, neurologic and cardiac signs often occur together in pediatric patients.

Neurologic Toxicity

Intravascular Injection

In case of accidental intravascular injection, the symptoms of neurologic toxicity of a LA are: a brisk headache, a metallic taste in the mouth, numbness or tingling of the lips, irritability, restlessness, blurred vision. With further increases in plasma concentration, convulsions occur. At very high plasma concentrations, LA produce burst suppression and electrical silence on the EEG. Before the injection, the awake and cooperative patient should be warned to inform the practitioner if she or he experiences those symptoms during or shortly after it; this is obviously difficult to obtain in young children. Verbal contact (i.e., making the child talk during the injection) should thus be maintained with the child in order to detect these symptoms and signs as quickly as possible.

Overdose

In case of overdose (e.g., during the continuous infusion of a LA solution or following the administration of an excessive dose of the LA), the early signs of toxicity are less obvious because the blood levels raise more slowly: the possibility of ongoing neurologic toxicity should be borne in mind when the child presents with somnolence or agitation, jitteriness, tremulations, myoclonias, or of course, convulsions.

Treatment of Systemic Neurologic Toxicity

The clinical context in which the convulsions occur is important because those caused by accidental intravascular injection usually terminate within one or two

Table 2 Symptomatic Treatment of Local Anesthetic Toxicity

In case of	
- signs of central nervous system irritability (agitation, jitteriness, tremulations)	⇒ stop the injection administer pure oxygen hyperventilate the child if he or she is unconscious
- seizures	
- modification of the EKG trace (if available)	
- cardiac dysrhythmias	
If seizures persist	⇒ diazepam 0.1–0.5 mg/kg IR or IV or midazolam 0.05–0.1 mg/kg IV or IM or propofol 2 mg/kg IV or thiopental 2–4 mg/kg IV *If the above treatment fails*: endotracheal intubation and curarisation
In case of cardiovascular collapse or arrest	⇒ external cardiac massage and ACLS according to EKG trace
	⇒ IV administration of Intralipid [R]: 1 mL/kg in 1 min to be repeated twice at 3–5 min interval and converted to an infusion at a rate of 0.25 mL/kg/min until hemodynamic stability is restored[a]

[a]Dosage inferred from adult data.

minutes because the blood concentration of LA decreases quickly by redistribution. On the contrary, convulsions caused by overdose may be prolonged and more difficult to treat because hepatic drug metabolism is required to reduce the blood concentration of LA (14). The treatment is summarized in Table 2. When caring for a child presenting with neurologic signs of LA toxicity, one should carefully titrate the anticonvulsant drugs used bearing in mind that the child's heart is in a vulnerable state and probably on the verge of cardiac involvement.

Cardiovascular Toxicity

The signs of cardiovascular toxicity are well described for racemic bupivacaine; an increase in PR interval and major widening of QRS usually precede arrhythmias (ventricular tachycardia, rarely torsades de pointe) that are followed, if the administration of the LA is not interrupted, by either ventricular fibrillation or profound bradycardia heralding cardiac arrest with asystole.

Both clinically and experimentally, the signs of cardiovascular toxicity of the other amide LA (especially the most recent ones such as ropivacaine and levobupivacaine) are similar but occur at higher blood concentrations and are easier to treat.

Table 3 Maximal Doses of Local Anesthetics in Children (in mg/kg)

	Without epinephrine	With epinephrine
Procaine	7	10
Chloroprocaine	10	20
Tetracaine (Amethocaine)	1.5	1 (?)
Lidocaine	5	7
Prilocaine	5	7
Mepivacaine	5	7
Bupivacaine	2.5	3
Levobupivacaine	2.5 (?)	3 (?)
Ropivacaine	3	?

Source: From Ref. 80.

Prevention of Toxicity

The first step is to know the child's medical history, allergies and body weight.

Before using an LA solution, the practitioner needs to calculate the maximum dose and volume that can be administered to the patient (Table 3), knowing that a 1% solution contains 10 mg/mL.

In case of injection of an LA, the equipment for immediate resuscitation in case of systemic reaction (face mask, source of oxygen, Ambu® bag to support ventilation) should be checked and ready for use. Moreover, before and during the injection of the solution, an aspiration test should be performed in order to avoid accidental intravascular injection; this test is however fallible because of the small size of the vessels and vigilance is mandatory. If a locoregional block (e.g., femoral nerve or caudal block) is performed in a sedated or anesthetized child, most anesthesiologists add some epinephrine (1/200,00 or 1/400,000) to the LA solution: this is called a test dose and produces early electrocardiographic and hemodynamic effects (change in T-wave size, increase in heart rate) in case of intravascular injection. During the injection in an awake child, the practitioner should maintain verbal contact with the child in order to detect as quickly as possible discrete symptoms and signs of neurologic toxicity (bad taste in the mouth, agitation, and logorrhea). Any abnormal physical or behavioral reaction must lead to immediate interruption of the injection and the clinical evaluation of the patient.

Last, the patient should be monitored during at least 30 minutes after the injection because, depending on the route of administration of the LA, peak systemic concentrations occur within 15 to 45 minutes after the injection.

Treatment of Toxic Reactions

It should be borne in mind that not every reaction occurring during the use of a LA is caused by its systemic resorption: either a vasovagal (bradycardia, sudation, palor) or an allergic reaction (rash, hypotension, bronchospasm) can also occur and they should be diagnosed and treated appropriately.

In case of toxic reaction during or following the use of LA, the treatment principles are to ensure the child's oxygenation, to prevent the development of respiratory acidosis and, if necessary, to apply the rules of pediatric cardiac life support. Some authors advise against the use of epinephrine during cardiovascular resuscitation in case of bupivacaine intoxication because it produces tachycardia and could favor dysrhythmias: epinephrine is however still useful in those circumstances but IV bolus doses not greater than 5 a 10 µg/kg should be used. In animal models and in a few adult case reports, the rapid IV administration of a 20% lipid solution (Intralipid ^{R}) has been successfully used in case of acute cardiac toxicity of a LA, but no experience in children has been published so far (15). A stepwise approach of the treatment of symptoms of LA intoxication, including a proposed dosage for Intralipid administration as inferred from the experience in adults, is proposed in Table 2.

LOCAL ANESTHESIA IN PEDIATRIC DERMATOLOGIC SURGERY

Pain Assessment in Children

The goal of pain assessment is to provide as objective as possible data to determine which actions should be taken to alleviate or abolish the child's pain and to evaluate their effectiveness. Producing a cooperative child is an insufficient goal if the child suffers "in silence." Pain can be evaluated by observing behavior (what children do), measuring biological markers (how their bodies react) and self-report (what children say).

Physiological measures have been used to evaluate pain associated with short-term medical procedures but reveal more the importance of the stress reaction than pain intensity. Therefore, behavioral pain scales have to be considered.

In the recent years, patterns of behavior (facial expression, body/limb movements and crying) have been increasingly studied. In neonates and small infants, pain-associated facial expressions allowed the development of so-called facial coding systems, such as the NFCS (Neonatal Facial Coding System) (16). Body movement in response to a painful stimulus can be used to assess pain in the preverbal child, but lack of movement does not always indicate the absence of pain; it may indicate a very high level of pain. Preschool children usually lack the verbal and cognitive skills to describe their feelings of pain or physical discomfort. Many creative tools have been developed to help them indicate the degree of their pain. Examples are drawings of faces, a photographic scale of facial expression, and a ladder scale. To help the care provider, many multidimensional composite measures have been developed such as: CHEOPS (17), TPPPS (18), and COMFORT (19). For older children and adolescents, visual analogue scales (VAS) have been shown to be reliable for pain measurement.

Topical Anesthesia of Intact Skin

Children who need painful dermatologic procedures should benefit from one of the several excellent, noninvasive anesthetics and delivery systems that are available. The routine and appropriate use of topical anesthetic agents is comforting not only to young patients, but also to families and pediatric practitioners. The characteristics of the topical anesthetic used must be adapted to the foreseen procedure. Will the produced analgesia be sufficient or partial? In the first case, the appropriate dose and application time should be used in order to reduce the incidence of adverse events. In the second case, it should be decide if topical anesthesia will be used as a "premedication" before a local infiltration or if sedation will be associated.

EMLA

EMLA (acronym for eutectic mixture of local anesthetics) cream is an oil-in-water emulsion containing 2.5% lidocaine and 2.5% prilocaine. Since this agent is extensively described in chapter 4 (Topical anesthesia), only pediatric data will be reviewed hereafter. In adults, depth and duration of analgesia is dependant on the application time, but the maximum depth of kin anesthesia obtainable is 5 mm (20). Although it has not been studied in children, similar results can be expected: their skin is thinner, possibly leading to a greater diffusion distance, but the cutaneous blood flow is higher, decreasing the depth and duration of anesthesia by a washout effect.

Modes of application. EMLA has to be applied under an occlusive dressing (e.g., Tegaderm, Micropore®) but, in neonates, ordinary cellophane can be used reducing pain and risk of skin damage at removal (21). Considering age and weight, strict guidelines regarding maximal total dose, application area and application times of EMLA on intact skin are listed on Table 4. Shorter application times are indicated for

Table 4 Recommended EMLA® Dosing on Intact and Healthy Skin in Children

Age and body weight	Maximum total dose (g)	Maximum application area (cm^2)	Maximum application time (hr)
0–3 mo or <5 kg	1	10	1
2–12 mo and >5 kg	2	20	4
1–6 yr and >10 kg	10	100	4
7–12 yr and >20 kg	20	200	4

Table 5 Major Dermatologic Indications in Children and the Recommended
Application Times for EMLA[R]

Indications	Application times (min)
Curettage *Molluscum contagiosum*	30–60 (15 in atopic dermatitis)
Skin biopsy (pretreatment before skin infiltration)	60–120
Cauterization condylomata acuminate	5–15
Pulsed-dye laser (Port-wine stains)	60 (+ additional sedation?)
Minor tissue debridement	30
Vaccination	60

disease-affected skin, genital sites, and oral mucosa, because of the more rapid rate of
LA absorption from these locations. For small application areas, a tick layer is more
efficient than a thin one. Skin pigmentation does not affect the efficacy of EMLA
cream (22).

Often used to facilitate outpatient dermatologic procedures, the parental
application of EMLA has been shown to be no less effective than application by
trained medical personnel (23). A recent case report of development of seizures
after a parental application of a proper amount of EMLA but applied to a large
area of diseased skin, highlight the necessity to provide precise information to
the parents (amount, application area and timing) (24). If possible (i.e., skin
surface less than 10 cm^2), the use of an EMLA patch is therefore advised.

Adequacy of analgesia. Venipuncture and venous cannulation are the most
studied indications in the literature. Even in these cases, great variations of
success rate are observed (25–27). The most relevant factors related to EMLA
efficacy are type of procedure, duration of application, and the child's anxiety (28).
Several dermatologic indications are described below; the major ones are listed
on Table 5, with their respective recommended application times.

>   Curettage of *Molluscum contagiosum*: An application time of 30 to
>   60 minutes seems sufficient to produce good analgesia (no pain or
>   only slight pain) in children (29,30). A shorter application time
>   (15–30 minutes) has been proven sufficient and safe in children
>   with atopic dermatitis (31). As often multiple lesions are simultaneously
>   treated, attention should be paid to total dose and application area.
>   *Skin biopsy*: Despite topical anesthesia, deep pain is often reported.
>   An EMLA patch should therefore be used as local "premedication"
>   60 minutes before a slow subcutaneous infiltration with lidocaine (32).
>   *Cauterization or laser treatment of condylomata acuminate (CA)*: More
>   frequent in adults and adolescents, CA have also been seen in
>   children. Anesthesia of vulval and anal mucosa occurs after very

short application times (5–15 minutes) of EMLA cream. Longer application times are potentially toxic (rapid systemic resorption by the mucous membranes), and even resulted in less effective analgesia (33).

Pulsed-dye laser (port-wine stains): EMLA cream does not affect the degree of lightening of port-wine stain achieved during treatment and can thus be used in children. However, although good results have been described (34), anxiety seems to play an important role during these repeated procedures in which immobility is mandatory. The use of additional sedation (see section "Tumescent Anesthesia") or the choice for short general anesthesia seems less traumatic, especially in young children.

Minor tissue debridement or laceration suture: although not recommended by the manufacturer, EMLA cream has been used in open wound with good results (35). In that study, low dose of EMLA (0.15 g/kg to max 5g total dose) was safe and more effective than TAC (see repair of lacerations).

Intramuscular or subcutaneous injection: The usefulness of EMLA before vaccination remains controversial (36) because the pain of subcutaneous or intramuscular injection occurs not only upon skin penetration but also during the injection in the subcutaneous or intramuscular space (tissue stretching, effect of pH and composition of the injectate).

Cryotherapy of common warts: EMLA does not penetrate the highly hyperkeratotic wart area at a rate sufficient to allow accumulation of LA in the skin, and does not provide sufficient analgesia (37).

Adverse events. The most commonly observed side effects of EMLA are minor and consist of local blanching or erythema.

One of the most serious complications of the use of EMLA is methemoglobinemia. Signs include pallor and mottling of the skin, perioral cyanosis, and evidence of poor peripheral perfusion: it can occur even hours after the removal of EMLA cream from the skin (38). Infants zero to three months of age are at increased risk for it because prilocaine is metabolized in methemoglobinemia-producing agents and they have lower levels of erythrocyte methemoglobin reductase than adults (7). In the cases published the associated causal factors were: a too large amount applied, a too long application time or the coadministration of other methemoglobinemia-inducing agents such as sulfonamide derivates, acetaminophen, metoclopramide. In neonates and small infants, EMLA cream should be applied in smaller amounts and with a shorter application time, as recommended in Table 4.

Another potential toxicity of EMLA is systemic intoxication. A few cases of seizures after EMLA application are described in the literature (24,39). Most occurred when the maximum total dose, the maximum application area and/or time—according to the patient's age—were not respected in the presence of diseased skin.

A few purpuric reactions have been described after EMLA application (40,41). Purpura may be more common in premature infants and in patients with atopic dermatitis. Since these reactions could not be reproduced upon patch testing, it was advocated that the underlying mechanism was toxic rather than allergic (42). Complete resolution of that phenomenon was observed after a few days.

Eyelid applications should be performed with great caution: corneal deepithelializations (even requiring a corneal graft) have been described after inadvertent direct contact of EMLA with the cornea (43).

ELA-max [R]

ELA-max, a more recent development in topical anesthesia, contains 4% or 5% (ELA-max5) lidocaine encapsulated in a liposomal vehicle. In comparative clinical studies, ELA-max and EMLA were equally effective in reducing the pain associated with superficial surgical interventions. The liposomal delivery system of ELA-max increases the concentration and the residence time of the drug in the dermis and epidermis, and produces a longer duration of analgesia (44,45). Different studies compared the efficacy of ELA-max and EMLA in reducing the pain of venipuncture in children. Using a 100 mm visual analogue scale and observed behavioral distress scores to assess the level of associated pain, the data revealed no statistically significant difference in efficacy between a 60-minute EMLA application under occlusion and a 30-minute ELA-max application without occlusion (46,47). The apparent faster onset of anesthesia is a significant advantage in clinical practice. There have been no reports yet of serious adverse effects with the use of ELA-max. The absence of prilocaine suppresses the risk of methemoglobinemia as associated with the use of EMLA in infants. Although lidocaine toxicity has not been reported with ELA-max, caution should be exercised when applying ELA-max over large areas for more than two hours. The amount of lidocaine systemically absorbed is directly related to both the duration of application and the surface area to which it is applied. ELA-max is not recommended on mucous membranes. In children weighing less than 20 kg, a single application of ELA-max cream should not be applied to an area larger than 100 cm^2 (48). The safety and efficacy of ELA-max for dermatologic procedures in infants and children should be further investigated, including studies of minimal application times and the possible influence of an occlusive dressing on the time course of cutaneous anesthesia.

Tetracaine Formulations Used on Intact Skin

Amethocaine [R] is a 4% tetracaine gel preparation with a quicker onset and longer duration of action than EMLA cream (49,50). In 148 children, 1.5 g Amethocaine gel produced satisfactory reduction of pain for venous cannulation in 92%

of the cases after an application time of 40 minutes, with no significant adverse effects (51). A recent Cochrane meta-analyze shows that Amethocaine was even superior to EMLA regardless of whether application time was short (30–60 minutes) or long (more than 60 minutes) (52). Another advantage is that Amethocaine gel provides vasodilatation instead of vasoconstriction as EMLA usually does: this should facilitate venous puncture but has not be proven yet (53,54). It might also be superior to EMLA in reducing the pain of the flash lamp pulsed-dye laser treatment of port-wine stains in children (55).

Local effects include transient erythema, edema, urticaria, and pruritus. Site of application and age seems to be important factors in the occurrence of local reactions (56). In that study, the urticarial reaction was 10 times more frequent when the product was applied at the antecubital fossa compared with the dorsum of the hand. Urticarial reaction was also much more frequent in younger children (less than 4 years old) in comparison with older children.

As it does not expose the patient to a risk of methemoglobinemia (it contains no prilocaine), Amethocaine gel has been evaluated for procedural pain in neonates. Jain showed an analgesic effect of Amethocaine after a 30-minute application time; moreover, although the analgesia was not significantly higher after 60-minute application, the duration of effect was 3 hours instead of 1.5 hours (57). Other studies failed to show such an analgesic effect in neonates (58). A novel tetracaine patch on trial offers the double advantage that a specific amount of drug is delivered into a specific skin area and that its improved adhesive properties cause no trauma to the delicate skin of the neonate (5).

Tetracaine has a low bioavailability when applied topically on intact skin. The clinician should be aware of the increased risk of allergic reactions with the use of ester LA as compared with amide LA.

The use of liposome-encapsuled tetracaine (LET) has not been studied in the pediatric population, but in adult clinical trials, LET appears to be more effective than EMLA for venipuncture after a 60-minute application time (59).

Other Topical Anesthetics

The S-Caine Patch® contains a 1:1 eutectic mixture of lidocaine (70 mg) and tetracaine (70 mg). The system generates a controlled level of heating (39–41°C), which accelerates transcutaneous delivery of the LA, reducing by this way the analgesia onset time. A 20-minute application time seems to be sufficient for venous puncture in children without causing significantly more local adverse reaction compared with a placebo patch (60).

Betacaine-LA® ointment is a newly formulated topical anesthetic containing lidocaine, prilocaine, and a vasoconstrictor. The exact concentrations of its ingredients are a trade secret (61). The manufacturer reports concentrations of lidocaine and prilocaine to be four times greater that those found in EMLA. Its use is not recommended in children.

Topicaine[R] is 4% lidocaine in a gel microemulsion drug delivery system. Topicaine is approved for the temporary relief of pain and itching on normal skin. The recommended application time is 30 to 60 minutes and the maximum area of application in children should be 100 cm^2 (62). But as data regarding the percutaneous absorption of this preparation of lidocaine are not yet available in children, its use cannot be recommended for this population.

Topical Anesthesia for Repair of Lacerations

When facing the repair of a skin laceration in a child, we have first to answer the following questions:

1. Does this lesion really need a surgical suture? Are alternative solutions usable such as application of biological glue or use of Steri-Strips[R]?
2. If it has to be sutured, is the extent of tissue damage compatible with the use of a nontoxic dose of LA?
3. Will the operating conditions be comfortable and safe for both the child and for the practitioner?

Moreover, the choice for the most adapted technique of anesthesia (topical anesthesia, local infiltration, associated sedation or general anesthesia) depends also on the child's age and ability to cooperate.

The topical anesthetic combination of 0.5% tetracaine, 1:1000 epinephrine, and 11.8% cocaine (TAC) is a useful preparation for the exploration and repair of lacerations. With this composition, the maximal dose recommended in children is 0.05 mL/kg. TAC formulations, as well as the newer formulations, are more effective on the face and scalp than on the extremities. Extensive absorption of cocaine from mucous membranes has been associated with seizures (63,64) and death (65). A preparation less concentrated in cocaine (4.0%) has been shown to be as effective as the classic TAC preparation for children's face and scalp lacerations sutures (66), and is thus safer.

Formulations substituting lidocaine for cocaine (e.g., LAT: lidocaine 4%, epinephrine 1:1000 and tetracaine 0.5%) are effective for laceration repair and may be preferable to TAC preparations to avoid the risks and administrative problems associated with the use of cocaine (67,68).

EMLA, however not recommended for this application, appears to be superior to TAC for anesthesia of simple extremity lacerations in children (35). Specific protocols should be developed to allow efficient use of EMLA in these indications.

Smith et al. compared different non-cocaine-containing LA solutions in the pediatric populations (69–71). In their experience, the association of bupivacaine 0.48% and norepinephrine 1:26,000 is very effective. Whether, in this indication, ropivacaine or levobupivacaine (the new less cardiotoxic LA) will be as effective as bupivacaine is open to investigation.

Because of the problem of storing cocaine amounts into the Emergency Department, only few European departments use TAC solutions. In our institution, we obtain good results with a home-made lidocaine 4% gel with epinephrine (lidocaine 40 mg, epinephrine 1:200,000, propylene glycol gel ad 1 mL).

Topical Anesthesia of Mucosal Surfaces

Viscous lidocaine, cetacaine, benzocaine, and EMLA with or without occlusion have all proven to be effective local agents for reducing the pain of lidocaine infiltration and during superficial procedures, including cryotherapy of mucosal lesions (72). In infants, the use of cetacaine and benzocaine is contraindicated because of the risk of methemoglobinemia (73).

Viscous lidocaine 2% provides analgesia after an application time of 5 to 10 minutes, and it lasts for 20 to 30 minutes. For mucosal application, the maximal dose of lidocaine is 3 mg/kg in children and 2 mg/kg under three years of age. If repeated applications are needed, the maximum dose of lidocaine is 2 mg/kg per hour. Moreover, attention should be paid to the risk of large resorption by inflammed mucosae (e.g., mucositis) and the risk of aerodigestive tract anesthesia if the solution is swallowed by the child. Cases of accidental intoxication after prescription or administration errors are unfortunately still occurring (74).

Infiltration Anesthesia

Selection of the Local Anesthetic

To optimize the risk-benefit ratio of using infiltration anesthesia in pediatric patients, it is critical to emphasize two general principles. The *first* is familiarity with the properties and dosage limits of the LA to be used: using an unfamiliar LA increases the risk of dosage or concentration errors. After having calculated the maximum dose and volume that can be administered to the patient, the practitioner needs to evaluate if they are compatible with the surface area to be infiltrated. This is essential in cases of large skin lacerations, where general anesthesia sometimes offers more comfort and security to the child and better working conditions to the doctor. The *second* is the selection of LA whose duration of action is appropriate to the desired effect so that a single-injection technique can be used. Short acting LA (e.g., lidocaine), offering a rapid onset, are used for short procedures after which minimal postoperative pain is expected. For longer procedures, the use of long acting LA, despite their slower onset, provides good early postoperative analgesia. Mixing two LA, in order to compensate the aforementioned limitations (slow onset/short duration), remains controversial. The toxicities of amide LA are not independent and should instead be considered additive (75). When LA are combined, the maximum dose of each should be adjusted in proportion; thus, if the first LA is given at one-half of its maximum recommended dose, the second should be administered at no more than one-half of its own recommended maximum dose.

Epinephrine, the most commonly used adjuvant, has been described earlier (see section "Epinephrine")

Technique for Local Infiltration in Awake Children

The goals are to reduce the child's pain and stress and to obtain good working conditions for the practitioner: a calm immobile child allows a rapid and precise surgery. Moreover, this medical experience should be made as positive as possible to the child in order to make a positive life experience of it (sense of pride) and to avoid future phobic reactions directed to nonpainful stimuli (entering the hospital, visiting a doctor). A few tricks can be used to give the technique the best chances of success (76):

- Be calm, create a relaxed atmosphere, and be devoted to this task (avoid interruptions by beeper, phone calls, etc.).
- Encourage parental presence. The parents' role is to encourage, and not to restrain the child!
- Prepare the equipment (needles, syringes, etc.) out of the eyesight of the child.
- If possible (on intact skin), use topical anesthesia (e.g., EMLA) as "premedication" 60 minutes before introducing the infiltration needle.
- Explain to the child the sensations he or she will experience during the infiltration (pinching, transient burning sensation during injection, etc.) and the fact that afterward some nonpainful sensations will remain (feeling that something is done, but no pain). Promising to a child that "you won't feel anything" exposes to a risk of panic reactions (the child thinks the technique has failed because he or she still feels something), and thus of failure.
- Encourage the active participation of the child: "Take a deep breath, good . . . breathe slowly now and try to relax, good . . . it helps me a lot . . ."
- Use small needles (22–25 gauge).
- Warming the used LA to body temperature can reduce pain (77).
- Buffering the LA solutions with sodium bicarbonate significantly reduces pain on injection. By adding 1 mL of sodium bicarbonate 8.4% to 9 mL of lidocaine, the solution is brought to a physiologic pH, which reduces injection pain. Buffered solutions (especially adrenaline-containing solutions) need conservation at 4°C in closed containers for storage.
- Injecting the first milliliters as slowly as possible is another efficient way to reduce pain (78). Subcutaneous injection has a slower onset but is less painful than intradermal injection.
- Wait at least 5 minutes (after lidocaine, mepivacaine) or 15 minutes (after bupivacaine, ropivacaine) before proceeding. By doing this, you respect

the onset time of the LA. Most failures are due to the impatience of the practitioner!

- Do not persist in case of failure. Renegotiate with the child, or change for another technique.
- Do not forget to congratulate the child at the end.

Iontophoresis

Iontophoresis is a transdermal drug delivery system that uses an electric current to carry ionized lidocaine through the stratum corneum (79). Drug delivery is proportional to the product of the strength and duration of the current (mA/min). Some interesting pediatric points are highlighted here, but for general information about this system, we recommend the reader to go to chapter 9.

Most school-age children will be fascinated by this method of drug delivery and will accept the itching, tingling, or warmth sensations it produces. In younger children, individual anxiety level should be assessed first. If the child does not complete the 10 to 15 minutes application time, a rescue technique will be required and this delay (and maybe a painful infiltration) may, in comparison with parental application of EMLA at home, result in dissatisfaction of the patient, the parent, and other healthcare workers. Most studies have used 30 to 40 mA·min as a standard iontophoretic dose, but the use of a smaller dose, in anxious children, may improve the tolerability and still be efficacious (80,81). While the efficacy and safety of lidocaine iontophoresis for IV cannulation in pediatric patients has been demonstrated in open (81,82), comparative (e.g., versus EMLA) (83,84), and placebo-controlled (85) clinical trials, the studies evaluating its efficacy for dermatologic procedures include only a few number of patients. Lidocaine iontopheresis providing deeper anesthesia than EMLA (up to 10 mm deep), can be advantageous for procedures such as skin biopsies, where supplemental local anesthetic infiltration, often needed with topical anesthetics, can cause tissue distortion. New easy-to-use and well-tolerated disposable lidocaine delivery systems have recently been developed and seem to provide local anesthesia with a much shorter onset (2–3 minutes) (86).

The inability to anesthetize a large area or to cover more than one site with iontophoresis is a limiting factor. A few cases of burns (incidence of 1:10,000 to 1:20,000 treatments) due to defective equipment have been described. An effort should be made to define the minimal effective time-current product needed for dermatologic procedures in children so as to minimize the adverse events and maximize the tolerability of the technique.

Tumescent Anesthesia

For the full description of this technique, we send the reader to chapter 7. Many issues need to be addressed before tumescent local anesthesia is routinely incorporated into pediatric dermatologic surgery. Very high doses of lidocaine (up to 50 mg/kg) are used for liposuccion in the adult awake patient. This is obviously not recommended in awake sedated or anesthetized children. LA have different pharmacologic properties in children, and they are not sucked up during the procedure as during liposuccion in adults. Bussolin et al. (87) showed that low-dosage tumescent local anesthesia (lidocaine maximum dose of 7 mg/kg with sodium bicarbonate in lactated Ringer's solution and 1:1,000,000 epinephrine), in combination with general anesthesia, seems to be a safe anesthesia technique for the surgical treatment of noncontiguous burns in pediatric patients and that it offers prolonged postoperative analgesia. When a peripheral nerve block (which requires a lower dose of LA) is not possible, this can be an elegant technique under some conditions. In infants and young children, the solution has to be warmed at 37°C to decrease risk of inducing hypothermia, and the fluids administrated intravenously should be calculated with the fluid administered subcutaneously in order to minimize risk of fluid overload. The use of ropivacaine (long acting but less toxic than bupivacaine) will maybe become an attractive alternative to lidocaine or prilocaine in order to provide longer lasting postoperative analgesia (88), but more information is still needed in children.

Moehrle and Breuminger (89) used a slow injection infusion pump with success for tumescent local anesthesia in awake children older than six years of age. But no objective pain and behavioral measurement were utilized, making it difficult to assess the efficacy, the tolerability and thus the utility of this technique as compared to traditional techniques. Tumescent lidocaine anesthesia above the clavicle (head and neck) results in a higher and more rapid rise in plasma concentration when compared with lower injection and should be performed very carefully in children (90). The safety of this technique remains thus to be carefully assessed in pediatric patients (91).

Peripheral Nerve Blocks

Techniques of regional anesthesia are mainly used in pediatric patients as tools for relieving surgical or traumatic pain and improving postoperative comfort. Therefore, they should be seen as techniques of analgesia (and not anesthesia), in combination with deep sedation or light general anesthesia. Pediatric anesthesiologists, who routinely perform regional blocks in children and are trained to treat their possible complications, should be consulted when large dermatological or plastic surgery is planed in children. The indication for regional anesthesia is based on the evaluation of its benefit/risk ratio compared with the advantages and disadvantages of all other techniques of analgesia available, including parenteral narcotics. Several factors must be considered when making a decision about the most suitable regional block procedure for a particular case: the distribution of analgesia should cover the whole operative field and the risks of the anesthetic technique should be in balance with the importance of the surgical procedure. The selection of the LA to be used depends on its pharmacological properties, the site and duration of surgery, and the expected duration of postoperative pain. The use of continuous infusion catheters is, at the present time, the sole technique able to provide analgesia over 24 hours and permit daily wound care postoperatively. New long acting, less cardiotoxic molecules (as ropivacaine and levobupivacaine), will probably play a consistent role in the future.

Additional Sedation in Children

Although local anesthesia alone is effective for most dermatologic surgical procedures, it offers no relief from the significant anxiety that pediatric patients experience when facing a medical procedure. Despite the relaxed atmosphere obtained with behavioral management and the use of some cunning devices (e.g., the parent-child tent) (92), some children will need additional sedation. Guidelines for the proper use of sedative agents in pediatric patients have been published in 2006 (93). They outline in detail appropriate candidates for "minimal" (anxiolysis), "moderate" (frequently called "conscious sedation"), and "deep" sedation. It also clearly stated that any patient can readily progress from one level of sedation to another and that a designed individual other than the treating physician should be entrusted with the exclusive responsibility of ensuring the patient's safety. This includes the ability to monitor patient's consciousness, vital signs and airway maintenance, and to initiate resuscitation, should complications arise. The need for a systematic approach is strongly recommended and includes the following:

- the careful pre-sedation evaluation for underlying medical or surgical condition that would increase the risk from sedation
- an appropriate fasting time before any elective procedure
- a focused airway examination for enlarged tonsils or anatomic abnormalities that might increase the risk of upper airway obstruction regardless the sedative used (e.g., Down's syndrome). Respiratory compromise is more common in children who have enlarged tonsils, especially if there is a history of nocturnal snoring (94). Those cases should be taken in charge by an anesthesiologist.
- a clear understanding of the pharmacology of the medication(s) used and of their interactions
- a patient's chart containing a time-based record documenting the time, dosage, and effect of the administered drug(s)
- a properly equipped and staffed recovery area
- appropriate discharge instructions for the parents

Hereafter, we highlight two techniques (nitrous oxide and midazolam) that can be used by nonanesthesiologists with a good efficacy/safety ratio during pediatric dermatologic procedures. But the combination of these sedatives, their use in ill children or any other form of deep sedation, should be performed under the care of an anesthesiologist or a nurse anesthetist.

Nitrous Oxide

Nitrous oxide (N_2O) is a mildly potent inhalational agent that can reduce anxiety and provides sedation and superficial analgesia. It is actually the only form of conscious sedation achievable in children. Inhalation sedation with N_2O/O_2 is commonly used in dentistry and could be used in pediatric dermatologic surgery. Premixed 50% N_2O in oxygen administered by trained nurses has proved to be a

Table 6 Premixed N_2O/O_2 50/50 Inhalational Sedation: Advises for Use

1. Check the equipment before use
2. Prepare the child

- Create a relaxing atmosphere
- Present the mask and equipment; let him or her choose the color and the smell of it
- Describe the oncoming events
- Explain the possible feelings that will be experienced ("you'll feel strange," you'll feel like laughing")
- Do not promise, he or she will sleep.

3. Always associate local anesthesia

- Topical anesthesia or local infiltration

4. Do not apply the mask with force

- Try to reach "spontaneous acceptation" of the mask (a forced application will create agitation which will not be controlled by N_2O)

5. Encourage parental presence

- Is always helpful to limit the child's anxiety

6. Provide continuous inhalation

- Inhalational sedation has to be administered for at least 3 min before a painful stimulus
- A close-fitting mask should be applied: any leak will dilute the N_2O administered and thus reduce its efficacy
- Someone's attention should be kept on the child (a euphoric child can easily fall of the table)

7. To deal with an uncooperative child
Use smooth movement restriction during the start of inhalation (forced immobilization often creates additional agitation)

safe option for procedural sedation in children. In a prospective study of 35,828 administrations of 50% N_2O in O_2, among which 82% were in pediatric patients, 4.4% minor and 0.08% major complications were observed, respectively. Forty-five percent of the minor complications were nausea and vomiting; the remaining events were mainly euphoria or agitation. Among the major complications recorded, 12 were associated with coadministration of another sedative and 2 with bad monitoring of the patient. One case of laryngospasm occurred because a drowsy child vomited into the facemask, and one death was caused by hypoxia because the child was forced to inhale from an empty cylinder of gas (95).

Table 6 lists some practical points to be respected to obtain a high success rate with this technique. Contraindications to the use of N_2O nevertheless exist and are listed in Table 7.

Midazolam

Midazolam, a short-acting benzodiazepine, is a convenient sedative for procedures in children (96). This agent, not only alleviates anxiety, but induces anterograde conscious amnesia, making it particularly useful for procedures requiring multiple visits such as pulsed dye laser therapy for vascular anomalies (97). However, implicit or emotional memory is not affected by midazolam and

Table 7 Contraindication to the Use of Nitrous Oxide with Restricted Use for Non-Doctors

---

Absolute contraindication for administration of nitrous oxide:
Patients with:

- Intracranial hypertension
- Unconsciousness
- Pneumothorax
- Disorders involving accumulation of gas in closed body spaces (e.g. intestinal obstruction, chronic otitis media or sinusitis)
- Congenital or acquired (e.g., vegetarism) deficit in vitamin B_{12}, or conditions which can be worsened by decreased vitamin B_{12} availability (homocystinuria, tyrosinemia type I)

Contraindications for administration by non-doctors

- Children younger than 4 years (this threshold could be lowered to 1 year)
- Children on psychotropic drugs
- Children with an underlying condition that might impair respiratory or brain function

---

Source: From Ref. 99.

Table 8 Recommended Dosage of Midazolam and Their Advantages/Disadvantages According to the Route of Administration

Routes of administration	Recommended dose (mg/kg)	Advantage	Disadvantage
Oral	0.5–0.75	- Convenient administration - Onset 15 min	Unpleasant taste (use institution-made compositions or mix the IV solution with strawberry/ cherry elixir or acetaminophen syrup, or Versed[R] syrup)
Nasal	0.2	Rapid onset (5 min)	- Irritating - Not recommended
Rectal	0.3–0.5	- Useful in (uncooperative) young children - Onset 20–30 min	- Onset less predictable - Not always socially accepted
Intravenous	0.05–0.1	- Titration possible to achieve the level of sedation	- Intravenous access needed
Intramuscular	Not recommended		

could result in some postoperative behavioral problems. Midazolam has also no analgesic properties and should therefore always be associated with topical or local anesthesia. Although we recommend oral midazolam, it can be administered via other various routes which are described in Table 8.

The major concern with midazolam is respiratory depression, which may be life threatening, especially when used in association with other sedatives or with narcotics. Moreover, paradoxal reactions (agitation) are not uncommon as with any benzodiazepine (98).

CONCLUSION

When using local anesthesia to perform dermatological surgery in a child, selection of the most appropriate agent and technique is a matter of scientific knowledge, experience, and technical skills, but also of human compassion: case-by-case evaluation of what is best for a given child's physical and psychological comfort without jeopardizing safety is mandatory.

REFERENCES

1. Grunau RVE, Whitfield MF, Petrie JH. Pain sensitivity and temperament in extremely low-birth-weight premature toddlers and preterm and full-term controls. Pain 1994; 58:341–346.
2. Taddio A, Goldbach M, Ipp M, et al. Effect of neonatal circumcision on pain responses during vaccination in boys. Lancet 1994; 344:291–292.
3. Evans NJ, Rutter N. Development of the epidermis in the newborn. Biol Neonate 1986; 49:74–80.
4. Gourrier E, El Hanache A, Karoubi P, et al. Problèmes cutanés après application d'Emla[R] chez des prématurés. Arch Pediatr 1996; 3:289–290.
5. Long CP, McCafferty DF, Sittlington NM, et al. Randomized trial of novel tetracaine patch to provide local anesthesia in neonates undergoing venepuncture. Br J Anaesth 2003; 91:514–518.
6. Nilsson A, Engsberg G, Henneberg S, et al. Inverse relationship between age-dependent erythrocyte activity of methaemoglobin reductase and prilocaine-induced methaemoglobinaemia in infancy. Br J Anaesth 1990; 64:72–76.
7. Mazoit JX. Pharmacology of local anesthetics. In: Dalens B, Bissonnette B, eds. Pediatric Anesthesia: Principles and Practice. New York: Mc Graw-Hill, 2002:303–37.
8. Bachmann B, Biscoping J, Adams AA, et al. The importance of the site of blood sampling in determination of plasma concentrations of local anesthetics. Reg Anesth 1990; 13:16–20.
9. Mazoit JX, Denson DD, Samii K. Pharmacokinetics of bupivacaine following caudal anesthesia in infants. Anesthesiology 1988; 68:387–391.
10. Booker PD, Taylor C, Saba G. Perioperative changes in α 1-glycoprotein concentrations in infants undergoing major surgery. Br J Anaesth 1996; 76:365–368.
11. Meunier JF, Goujard E, Dubousset AM, et al. Pharmacokinetics of bupivacaine after continuous infusion in infants with and without biliary atresia. Anesthesiology 2001; 95:87–95.
12. Giaufre E, Bruguerolle B, Morrisson-Lacombe G, et al. The influence of midazolam on the plasma concentrations of bupivacaine and lidocaine after caudal injection of the mixture of the local anesthetics in children. Acta Anaesthesiol Scand 1990; 34:44–46.
13. Capron F, Perry D, Capolaghi B. Crise convulsive et methémoglobinémie après application de crème anesthésique (lettre). Arch Pediatr 1998; 5:812.
14. Rezvani M, Finkelstein Y, Verjee Z, et al. Generalized seizures following topical lidocaine administration during circumcision. Paediatr Drugs 2007; 9:125–127.
15. Rosenblatt MA, Abel M, Fisher GW, et al. Successful use of a 20% lipid emulsion to resuscitate a patient after a presumed bupivacaine related cardiac arrest. Anesthesiology 2006; 105:217–218.
16. Grunau RV, Craig KD. Pain expression in neonates: facial action and cry. Pain 1987; 28:395–410.
17. McGrath PJ, Johnson G, Goodman JT, et al. CHEOPS: a behavioral scale for rating postoperative pain in children. In: Fields L, Dubner R, Cervero F, eds. Advances in Pain Research and Therapy. New York: Raven Press, 1985:395–402.

18. Tarbell SE, Cohen IT, Marsh JL. The toddler-preschooler postoperative pain scale: an observational scale for measurement postoperative pain in children aged 1–5. Preliminary report. Pain 1992; 50:273–280.

19. Ambuel B, Hamlett KW, Marx CM, et al. Assessing distress in pediatric intensive care environments: the COMFORT scale. J Pediatr Psychol 1992; 17:95–109.

20. Bjerring P, Arendt-Nielsen L. Depth and duration of skin analgesia to needle insertion after topical application of EMLA cream. Br J Anaesth 1990; 64:173–177.

21. Gourrier E, Karoubi P, el Hanache A, et al. Use of EMLA® cream in a department of neonatology. Pain 1996; 68:431–434.

22. Riendeau LA, Bennett D, Black-Noller G, et al. Evaluation of the analgesic efficacy of EMLA® cream in volunteers with differing skin pigmentation undergoing venipuncture. Reg Anesth Pain Med 1999; 24:165–169.

23. Kou JL, Fanurik D, Stoner PD, et al. Efficacy of parental application of eutectic mixture of local anesthetics for intravenous insertion. Pediatrics 1999; 103:e79.

24. Parker JF, Vats A, Bauer G. EMLA toxicity after application for allergy skin testing. Pediatrics 2004; 113:410–411.

25. Cooper CM, Gerrish SP, Hardwick M, et al. EMLA cream reduces the pain of venepuncture in children. Eur J Anaesthiol 1987; 4:441–448.

26. Maunuksela E, Korpela R. Double-blinded evaluation of a lignocaine-prilocaine cream (EMLA) in children: effect on the pain associated with venous cannulation. Br J Anaesth 1986; 58:1242–1245.

27. Chang PC, Goresky GV, O'Connor G, et al. A multicentre randomized study of single-unit dose package of EMLA patch vs. EMLA 5% cream for venepuncture in children. Can J Anaesth 1994; 41:59–63.

28. Lander J, Hodgins M, Nazarali S, et al. Determinants of success and failure of EMLA®. Pain 1996; 64:89–97.

29. Rosdahl I, Edmar B, Gisslén H, et al. Curettage of *Molluscum contagiosum* in children: analgesia by topical application of lidocaine-prilocaine cream (EMLA®). Acta Derm Venereol (Stockh) 1988; 68:149–153.

30. De Waard-van der Spek FB, Orange AP, Lillieborg S, et al. Treatment of *Molluscum contagiosum* using a lidocaine/prilocaine cream (EMLA®) for analgesia. J Am Acad Dermatol 1990; 23:685–688.

31. Ronnerfalt L, Fransson J, Wahlgren CF. EMLA cream provides rapid pain relief for curettage of *Molluscum contagiosum* in children with atopic dermatitis without causing serious application-site reactions. Pediatr Dermatol 1998; 15:309–312.

32. De Waard-van der Spek FB, Mulder PGH, Orange AP. Prilocaine/lidocaine patch (EMLA®) as a local premedication for skin biopsy in children. J Am Acad Dermatol 1997; 37:418–421.

33. Ljunghall K, Lillieborg S. Local anesthesia with lidocaine/prilocaine cream (EMLA®) for cautery of condyloma acuminate on vulvar mucosa. The effect of timing of application of the cream. Acta Derm Venereol (Stockh) 1989; 69:362–365.

34. Tan OT, Stafford TJ. EMLA® for laser treatment of port-wine stains in children. Lasers Surg Med 1992; 12:543–548.

35. Zempsky WT, Karasic RB. EMLA versus TAC for topical anesthesia of extremity wounds in children. Ann Emerg Med 1997; 30:163–166.

36. De Waard-van der Spek FB, Bernsen JC, Mulder PGH, et al. EMLA® cream as a local anaesthetic in MMR vaccination. Int J Clin Pract 1998; 52:136.

37. Gupta AK, Koren G, Shear NH. A double-blind, randomized, placebo-controlled trial of eutectic lidocaine/prilocaine cream 5% (EMLA) for analgesia prior to cryotherapy of warts in children and adults. Pediatr Dermatol 1998; 15:129–133.

38. Frey B, Kehrer B. Toxic methaemoglobin concentrations in premature infants after application of a prilocaine-containing cream and peridural prilocaine. Eur J Pediatr 1999; 158:785–788.

39. Rincon E, Baker RL, Iglesias AJ, et al. CNS toxicity after topical application of EMLA cream on a toddler with *Molluscum contagiosum*. Pediatr Emerg Care 2000; 16:252–254.

40. Calobrisi SD, Drolet BA, Esterly NB. Petechial eruption after the application of EMLA® cream. Pediatrics 1998; 101:471–473.

41. Neri I, Savoia F, Guareschi E, et al. Purpura after application of EMLA cream in two children. Pediatr Dermatol 2005; 22:566–568.

42. De Waard-van der Spek FB, Orange AP. Purpura caused by EMLA® is of toxic origin. Contact Dermatitis 1997; 36:11–13.

43. Chevaleraud E, Leroy L, Lebuisson DA. Crème Emla: du bon usage des mises en garde. Ann Fr Anesth Reanim 1995; 14:459.

44. Bucalo BD, Mirikitani EJ, Moy RL. Comparison of skin anesthetic effect of liposomal lidicaine, nonliposomal lidocaine, and EMLA using 30-minute application time. Dermatol Surg 1998; 24:537–541.

45. Friedman PM, Fogelman JP, Nouri K, et al. Comparative study of the efficacy of four topical anesthetics. Dermatol Surg 1999; 25:950–954.

46. Eichenfield LF, Funk A, Fallon-Friedlander S, et al. A clinical study to evaluate the efficacy of ELA-max (4% liposomal lidocaine) as compared with EMLA cream for pain reduction of venipuncture in children. Pediatrics 2002; 109:1093–1099.

47. Koh J, Harrison D, Myers R, et al. A randomized, double-blind comparison study of Emla® and ELA-Max® for topical anesthesia in children undergoing intravenous insertion. Paediatr Anaesth 2004; 14:977–82.

48. ELA-max package insert. Ferndale, MI: Ferndale Laboratories, Inc., 1997.

49. Huang W, Vidimos A. Topical anesthetics in dermatology. J Am Acad Dermatol 2000; 43:286–298.

50. O'Brien L, Taddio A, Lyszkiewicz D, et al. A critical review of the topical local anesthetic amethocaine (Ametop™) for pediatric pain. Paediatr Drugs 2005; 7:41–54.

51. Lawson RA, Smart NG, Gudgeon AC, et al. Evaluation of an amethocaine gel preparation for percutaneous analgesia before venous cannulation in children. Br J Anaesth 1995; 75:282–285.

52. Lander JA, Weltman BJ, So SS. EMLA and Amethocaine for reduction of children's pain associated with needle insertion. Cochrane Database Syst Rev 2006; 3: CD004236.

53. Choy L, Collier J, Watson AR. Comparison of lignocaine-prilocaine cream and amethocaine gel for local analgesia before venepuncture in children. Acta Paediatr 1999; 88:961–964.

54. Rømsing J, Henneberg SW, Walter-Larsen S, et al. Tetracaine gel vs. EMLA cream for percutanuous anaesthesia in children. Br J Anaesth 1999; 82:637–638.

55. McCafferty DF, Woolfson AD, Handley J, et al. Effect of percutaneous local anaesthetics on pain reduction during pulse dye laser treatment of portwine stains. Br J Anaesth 1997; 78:286–289.

56. Proudfoot C, Gamble C. Site-specific skin reactions to amethocaine. Paediatr Nurs 2006; 18:26–28.
57. Jain A, Rutter N. Topical amethocaine gel in newborn infant: how soon does it work and how long does it last?Arch Dis Child Fetal Neonatal Ed 2000; 83:F211–F214.
58. Lemyre B, Hogan D, Gaboury I, et al. How effective is tetracaine 4% gel, before a venipuncture, in reducing procedural pain in infants: a randomized double-blind placebo controlled trial. BMC Pediatr 2007; 7:7–14.
59. Fisher R, Hung O, Mezei M, et al. Topical anaesthesia of intact skin: liposome-encapsulated tetracaine vs EMLA. Br J Anaesth 1998; 81:972–973.
60. Sethna N, Verghese S, Hannallah R, et al. A randomized controlled trial to evaluate S-Caine Patch™ for reducing pain associated with vascular access in children. Anesthesiology 2005; 102:403–408.
61. Friedman PM, Mafong EA, Friedman ES, et al. Topical anesthetics update: EMLA and beyond. Dermatol Surg 2001; 27:1019–1026.
62. Topicaine package insert. Mountain View, CA: ESBA Laboratories, 1997.
63. Tripton GA, DeWitt GW, Eisenstein SJ. Topical TAC (tetracaine, adrenaline, cocaine) solution for local anesthesia in children: prescribing inconsistency and acute toxicity. South Med J 1989; 82:1344–1346.
64. Daya MR, Burton BT, Schleiss MR, et al. Recurrent seizures following mucosal application of TAC. Ann Emerg Med 1988; 17:646–648.
65. Daily RH. Fatality secondary to misuse of TAC solution. Ann Emerg Med 1988; 17: 159–160.
66. Smith SM, Barry RC. A comparison of three formulation of TAC (tetracaine, adrenalin, cocaine) for anesthesia of minor lacerations in children. Pediatr Emerg Care 1990; 6:266–270.
67. Ernst AA, Marvez-Valls E, Nick TG, et al. Lidocaine adrenaline tetracaine gel versus tetracaine adrenaline cocaine gel for topical anesthesia in linear scalp and facial lacerations in children aged 5 to 17 years. Pediatrics 1995; 95:255–258.
68. White N, Kim M, Brousseau D, et al. The anesthetic effectiveness of lidocaine-adrenaline-tetracaine gel on finger lacerations. Pediatr Emerg Care 2004; 20: 812–815.
69. Smith GA, Strausbaugh SD, Harbeck-Weber C, et al. Prilocaine-phenylephrine and bupivacaine-phenylephrine topical anesthetics compared with tetracaine-adrenaline-cocaine during repair of laceration. Am J Emerg Med 1998; 16:121–124.
70. Smith GA, Strausbaugh SD, Harbeck-Weber C, et al. Comparison of topical anes-thetics without cocaine to tetracaine-adrenaline-cocaine and lidocaine infiltration during repair of laceration: bupivacaine-norepinephrine is an effective new topical anesthetic agent. Pediatrics 1996; 97:301–307.
71. Smith GA, Strausbaugh SD, Harbeck-Weber C, et al. New non-cocaine containing topical anesthetics compared with tetracaine-adrenaline-cocaine during repair of lacerations. Pediatrics 1997; 100:825–830.
72. Svensson P, Arendt-Nielsen L, Bjerring P, et al. Oral mucosal analgesia quantita-tively assessed by argon laser-induced thresholds and single-evoked vertex poten-tials. Anesth Pain Control Dent 1993; 2:154–161.
73. Vessely MB, Zitsch RP. Topical anesthetic-induced methemoglobinemia: a case report and review of the literature. Otolaryngol Head Neck Surg 1993; 108:763–767.
74. Gonalez del Rei J, Wason S, Druckenbrod RW. Lidocaine overdose: another pre-ventable case? Pediatr Emerg Care 1994; 10:344–345.

75. Berde C. Regional anesthesia in children: what have we learned? Anesth Analg 1996; 83:897–900.
76. Veyckemans F, Annequin D. Practical use of local anesthetics in children. Arch Pediatr 2001; 8:991–999. Review (French).
77. Bainbridge LC. Comparison of room temperature and body temperature local anaesthetic solutions. Br J Plast Surg 1991; 44:147–148.
78. Scarfone RJ, Jasani M, Gracely EJ. Pain of local anaesthetics: rate of administration and buffering. Ann Emerg Med 1998; 31:36–40.
79. Pasero C. Lidocaine iontophoresis for dermal procedure analgesia. J PeriAnesth Nurs 2006; 21:48–52.
80. Zempsky WT, Sullivan J, Paulson DM, et al. Evaluation of a low dose lidocaine iontophoresis system for topical anesthesia in adults and children: a randomized, controlled trial. Clin Ther 2004; 26:1110–1119.
81. Zempsky WT, Anand KJS, Sullivan KM, et al. Lidocaine iontophoresis for topical anesthesia before intravenous line placement in children. J Pediatr 1998; 132: 1061–1063.
82. Schultz AA, Strout TD, Jordan P, et al. Safety, tolerability, and efficacy of iontophoresis with lidocaine for dermal anesthesia in ED pediatric patients. J Emerg Nurs 2002; 28:289–296.
83. Galinkin JL, Rose JB, Harris K, et al. Lidocaine iontophoresis versus EMLA for IV placement in children. Anesth Analg 2002; 94:1484–1488.
84. Suire SJ, Kirchhoff KT, Hissong K. Comparing two methods of topical anesthesia used before intravenous cannulation in pediatric patients. J Pediatr Health Care 2000; 14:68–72.
85. Rose JB, Galinkin JL, Jantzen EC, et al. A study of lidocaine iontophoresis for pediatric venipuncture. Anesth Analg 2002; 94:867–871.
86. Migdal M, Chudzynska-Pomianowska E, Vause E, et al. Rapid, needle-free delivery of lidocaine for reducing the pain of venipuncture among pediatric subjects. Pediatrics 2005; 115:393–398.
87. Bussolin L, Busoni P, Giorgi L, et al. Tumescent local anesthesia for the surgerical treatment of burns and postburn sequelae in pediatric patients. Anesthesiology 2003; 99:1371–1375.
88. Breuninger H, Hobbach PS, Schimek F. Ropivacaine: an important anesthetic agent for slow infusion and other forms of tumescent anesthesia. Dermatolog Surg 1999; 25:799–802.
89. Moehrle M, Breuninger H. Dermatosurgery using subcutaneous infusion anesthesia with prilocaine and ropivacaine in children. Pediatr Dermatol 2001; 18:469–472.
90. Rubin JP, Xie Z, Davidson C, et al. Rapid absorption of tumescent lidocaine above the clavicules: a prospective clinical study. Plast Reconstr Surg 2005; 115: 1744–1751.
91. Bell C. Tumescent local anesthesia for the surgical treatment of burns and postburn sequelae in pediatric patients. Surv Anesthesiol 2004; 48:243–244.
92. Yoo SS, Liggett RN, Cohen AC. Use of parent-child tents in pediatric laser surgery. Dermatol Surg 2003; 29:399–401.
93. Coté CJ, Wilson S, the Work group on Sedation, American Academy of Pediatrics, Amercian Academy of Pediatric Dentistry. Guidelines for monitoring and management of pediatric patients during and after sedation for diagnostic and therapeutic procedures: an update. Pediatrics 2006; 11:2587–2602.

94. Litman RS, Kottra JA, Berkowitz RJ, et al. Upper airway obstruction during mid-azolam/nitrous oxide sedation in children with enlarged tonsils. Pediatr Dent 1998; 20:318–320.
95. Onody P, Gil P, Hennequin M. Safety of a 50% nitrous oxide–oxygen premix: a prospective survey with 35,828 data sheets. Drugs Saf 2006; 29:633–640.
96. Otley CC, Nguyen TH, Phillips PK. Anxiolysis with oral midazolam in pediatric patients undergoing dermatologic surgical procedures. J Am Acad Dermatol 2001; 45:105–108.
97. Chen BK, Eichenfield LF. Pediatric anesthesia in dermatologic surgery: when hand-holding is not enough. Dermatol Surg 2001; 27:1010–1018.
98. Golparvar M, Saghaei M, Sajedi P, et al. Paradoxical reaction following midazolam premedication in pediatric patients—a randomized placebo controlled trial of ket-amine for rapid tranquilization. Pediatr Anesth 2004; 14:924–930.
99. Gall O, Annequin D, Benoit G, et al. Adverse events of premixed nitrous oxide and oxygen for procedural sedation in children. Lancet 2001; 358:1514–1515.

8

Iontophoresis for Local Anesthesia

William T. Zempsky

*Connecticut Children's Medical Center and
University of Connecticut School of Medicine,
Hartford, Connecticut, U.S.A.*

INTRODUCTION

Lidocaine iontophoresis allows for the transfer of lidocaine into the skin under the influence of electric current to provide dermal anesthesia. Recent studies support the use of this technology for anesthesia prior to procedures such as venous access, injection, shave biopsy, and pulse dye laser therapy. This chapter will review the history, principles, and clinical use of lidocaine iontophoresis for dermatologic procedures.

HISTORY

Aetius, a Greek physician, was the first to demonstrate the use of electricity for medical purposes when he showed that the shock of the torpedo fish could be used to treat the symptoms of gout (1). In the mid-18th century, Verati likely first described the technique of iontophoresis (1). In the early 1900s, Leduc demonstrated that the effects of iontophoresis were due to the delivery of charged drugs through the skin under the influence of a like charged electrode (1).

The first clinical use of iontophoresis was described by Gibson and Cooke in 1959 (2). Pilocarpine iontophoresis was used to induce sweating, allowing the collection of sweat, and the measurement of sweat chloride. The "sweat test" is still used in the diagnostic testing for cystic fibrosis.

More recently, iontophoresis has become commonly used in rehabilitation medicine for the transdermal delivery of dexamethasone for inflammatory conditions. Lidocaine iontophoresis is becoming more popular for topical anesthesia prior to a variety of procedures such as venipuncture and injection and minor dermatologic procedures that will be considered in depth later in this chapter. On the horizon is the use of iontophoresis to enhance the transdermal delivery of opiates, hormones, ophthalmologic agents as well as agents for the treatment of migraine and Parkinson's disease.

PRINCIPLES

Iontophoresis is the introduction of ions of soluble salts into the skin and/or mucosal surfaces under the influence of electric current (3). An iontophoretic circuit requires the placement of oppositely charged electrodes onto the skin. With activation of electric current, electrons flow through the skin beneath one electrode, through interstitial fluids, and back through the skin at the opposite electrode. An appropriately charged drug ion will migrate along the same path. Thus, a positively charged drug (i.e., lidocaine) inserted into the reservoir at the anode (positive electrode) is repelled toward the cathode (negative electrode). Conversely, negatively charged drugs (i.e., dexamethasone) are placed at the cathode and repelled toward the anode (Fig. 1).

Drug delivery in iontophoresis is dependent on multiple factors. It is proportional to the total electric charge (3). Total charge is a product of current intensity and duration and measured in milliampere-minutes (mA·min) (3). Acceptable anesthesia with lidocaine can be achieved with a dose of 15 to 40 mA·min (4–6).

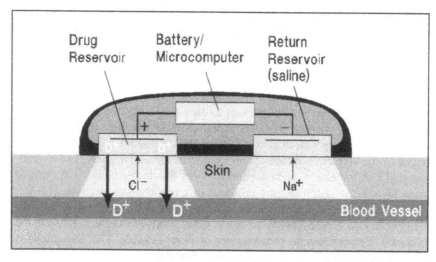

Figure 1 Schematic of iontophoretic circuit.

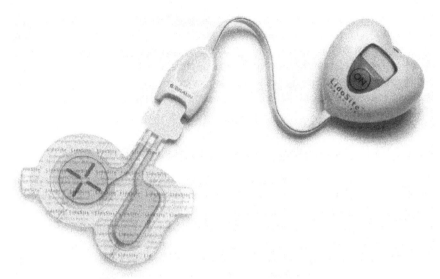

Figure 2 LidoSite™ lidocaine iontophoresis delivery system.

Transdermal iontophoresis is dependent on several drug-specific factors (7). The drug must be in an ionized state. The pH of the drug solution can be important if the degree of drug ionization is pH dependent. Drugs, which are more conductive, i.e., have a greater ability to allow transfer of electrical energy, are better candidates for iontophoretic delivery. Other ions of like charge in the selected drug in the iontophoretic solution may compete for the electrical current and make delivery less efficient. Transdermal delivery is inversely proportional to molecular weight and size.

Skin structure also exerts control over iontophoretic drug delivery (8). The stratum corneum is the principal barrier to electrical conductivity (9). Those areas of the body where stratum corneum is thicker, such as the palms and soles, are less conducive to iontophoretic drug delivery using currently available technology. The vascularity of the underlying skin also plays a role in iontophoretic drug delivery and efficacy. The areas with increased vascularity will allow more of the drug to be delivered systemically, and the local effects will be diminished.

An iontophoretic drug delivery system consists of a power source that provides electrical current, and two electrodes, a drug delivery electrode and a current return electrode. An example of a commercially available lidocaine iontophoresis system is LidoSite™ (Fig. 2). The LidoSite system contains a hydrogel drug delivery electrode that is impregnated with lidocaine. The current return electrode is located directly adjacent to the lidocaine electrode. The power source is reusable and attaches to the patch with a simple click mechanism. When the system is activated, lidocaine is delivered at a dose of 17 mA·min over a period of 10 minutes with automatic deactivation.

The likely principal mechanism for drug delivery in iontophoresis is electromigration (7). Ionic penetration likely occurs via aqueous pores, such as hair follicles and sweat ducts, as well as sebaceous glands and skin imperfections (10). Skin permeability may be altered by the application of electric current facilitating drug delivery. Finally, in some cases, electroosmosis may occur whereby the ions are carried across the skin in conjunction with the stimulation of osmotic flow (11).

LIDOCAINE IONTOPHORESIS: CLINICAL APPLICATIONS

Iontophoresis is an effective means to deliver lidocaine for topical anesthesia prior to procedures. In dermatology, superficial procedures such as shave biopsy, pulsed dye laser therapy, dermabrasion, and electrosurgery can be performed without additional anesthesia. For deeper procedures, lidocaine iontophoresis ameliorates or eliminates the pain associated with lidocaine infiltration.

The concentration of lidocaine used for iontophoresis usually varies between 1% and 4%. Iontophoresis with 2% lidocaine with epinephrine and 4% lidocaine with epinephrine provides equivalent anesthesia (12). It is likely that lidocaine concentration above a certain level does not affect anesthesia. In most cases, epinephrine is added to lidocaine for iontophoresis to prolong the duration of action by preventing vascular washout and systemic lidocaine absorption. In one study, the duration of anesthesia was lengthened from 12 to 87 minutes by the addition of 1:50,000 epinephrine to 4% lidocaine (13).

Lidocaine iontophoresis has several obvious advantages compared with lidocaine injection. While injection is effective and in many cases can be performed almost painlessly, it still requires a needle stick. In children, needle procedures can induce more fear than major surgical procedures and hospitalization. In adults "needle phobia" can result in significant anxiety and prevent them from undergoing important procedures. Lidocaine iontophoresis in contrast to injection can be performed without causing tissue distortion, thus simplifying many dermatologic procedures.

We have performed double-blind placebo-controlled studies of lidocaine iontophoresis for anesthesia prior to dermatologic procedures in both adults and children. Nineteen of 21 adults receiving shave biopsy after lidocaine iontophoresis required no supplemental anesthesia versus 2 of 20 adults receiving placebo ($p < 0.001$) (14). Twenty-nine of 31 children required no supplemental anesthesia for a range of procedures, including shave biopsy and curettage versus 2 of 29 placebo patients ($p < 0.001$) (6).

Lidocaine iontophoresis is also effective for anesthesia prior to pulsed dye laser treatment of port wine stains. Nunez evaluated 39 patients with port wine stains in a double-blind placebo-controlled study and found that lidocaine iontophoresis provided superior anesthesia to both placebo and mepivacaine (15). Kennard and Whitaker had similar findings in a comparison of lidocaine with placebo for anesthesia prior to laser therapy in 11 adults and children with port wine stains (16). Lidocaine iontophoresis has also been positively evaluated for anesthesia prior to cauterization of spider veins, abscess drainage, lesion excisions, and foreign-body removals (17,18).

Lidocaine iontophoresis is also very effective for topical anesthesia prior to venipuncture and intravenous access and has been compared with EMLA in this setting (4,5,19–22). Of four studies comparing lidocaine iontophoresis with EMLA, two found lidocaine iontophoresis to provide superior anesthesia, one found the two techniques to be equivalent, and one found EMLA to be superior (19–22). The study in which EMLA was superior utilized a lower iontophoretic dose than the other studies. Lidocaine iontophoresis has not been directly compared with EMLA for dermatologic procedures.

In choosing between these topical anesthetic methods, several factors should be weighed. Lidocaine iontophoresis can be accomplished in 10 minutes or less, while EMLA requires a 60-minute application time to be effective. Newer anesthetic creams such as LMX^4 require a 30-minute application. LMX^4 has not been compared directly to lidocaine iontophoresis but provides similar topical anesthesia to EMLA. Lidocaine iontophoresis provides anesthesia to a depth of 6 to 10 mm even at lower doses (23), while EMLA cream provides anesthesia to a maximal depth of 5 mm (24). This may be significant especially for more invasive dermatologic procedures. EMLA is preferable for procedures that cover a large area or for multiple simultaneous procedures. There are likely less side effects associated with EMLA use. The risks associated with iontophoretic drug delivery are discussed in the next section.

SAFETY

Lidocaine toxicity has not been reported during routine iontophoretic use. Ashburn found no detectable serum lidocaine in seven adults following iontophoresis with 2% lidocaine with 1:50,000 epinephrine at a dose of 40 mA·min at completion of iontophoresis and at 30, 60, and 120 minutes postiontophoresis (25). In a study of 12 children, only one had a detectable lidocaine level (8.9 ng/mL) following iontophoretic treatment (26). Therapeutic serum lidocaine levels range from 1500 to 5500 ng/mL, with toxic levels at above 6000 ng/mL (26).

Adverse effects from iontophoresis are predominately related to the iontophoretic current. They tend to be proportional to the total iontophoretic dose delivered and are more problematic at higher current levels. Many patients experience tingling, itching, or warmth during iontophoretic treatment. Erythema occurs after treatment often under the cathode for lidocaine iontophoresis. Urticaria secondary to mast cell activation can also be seen under the electrodes. Petechiae can also occur under the electrode placement areas. Occasionally, a patient will experience muscle spasm or parathesias during treatment, but these reactions resolve spontaneously. In our earlier study, about 5% of pediatric patients did not tolerate the electrical sensation associated with iontophoresis and asked that the treatment be terminated (4). This was not a problem in our recent study that utilized a lower total iontophoretic dose than previous studies, while not sacrificing efficacy (5).

The predominant concern regarding iontophoretic therapy is the potential for partial-thickness skin burns. Burns can be as small as a pinpoint and up to 5 mm in diameter. They can be caused by faulty electrode design, placement of electrodes over skin defects or other areas of low resistance, excessive current levels or iontophoretic dose, or the buildup of HCl or NaOH under the anode and cathode, respectively (27). The incidence of burns with iontophoretic therapy is reported to be between 1 in 10,000 and 1 in 20,000 treatments (28). Continued improvements in electrode design and sensors to recognize changes in skin resistance should alleviate this problem.

CONCLUSIONS

Lidocaine iontophoresis is an effective method for topical anesthesia prior to simple dermatologic procedures. It provides a rapid method to reduce the pain associated with these procedures in both adults and children.

REFERENCES

1. Li LC, Scudds RA. Iontophoresis: an overview of mechanisms and clinical applications. Arthritis Care Res 1995; 8:51–56.
2. Gibson LE, Cooke RE. A test for the concentration of electrolytes in sweat in cystic fibrosis of the pancreas utilizing pilocarpine by iontophoresis. Pediatrics 1959; 23:545–549.
3. Zempsky WT, Ashburn MA. Iontophoresis: noninvasive drug delivery. Am J Anesthesiol 1998; 25:158–162.
4. Zempsky WT, Anand KM, Sullivan KM, et al. Lidocaine iontophoresis for topical anesthesia prior to intravenous line placement in children. J Pediatr 1998; 132: 1061–1063.
5. Zempsky WT, Sullivan J, Paulson MD, et al. Evaluation of a low-dose iontophoresis system for topical anesthesia in adults and children: a randomized controlled trial. Clin Ther 2004; 26:1110–1119.
6. Zempsky WT, Parkinson TM. Lidocaine iontophoresis for topical anesthesia before dermatologic procedures in children: a randomized controlled trial. Pediatric Dermatol 2003; 20:364–368.
7. Banga AJ, Chien YW. Iontophoretic delivery of drugs: fundamentals, developments and biomedical applications. J Control Release 1988; 7:1–24.
8. Singh J, Maibach HI. Topical iontophoretic drug delivery in vivo: historical development, devices and future perspectives. Dermatology 1993; 187:234–238.
9. Singh S, Singh J. Transdermal drug delivery by passive diffusion and iontophoresis: a review. Med Res Rev 1993; 113:569–621.
10. Theib U, Kuhn I, Lucker PW. Iontophoresis—is there a future for clinical application? Methods Find Exp Clin Pharmacol 1991; 13:353–359.
11. Delgado-Charro MB, Guy RH: Characterization of convective flow during iontophoresis. Pharm Res 1994; 11:929–937.

12. Gagranosa LP. Defining a practical solution for iontophoretic local anesthesia of the skin. Methods Find Exp Clin Pharmacol 1981; 3(2):83–94.
13. Maloney JM, Bezzant JL, Stephen RL, et al. Iontophoretic administration of lidocaine anesthesia in office practice: an appraisal. J Dermatol Surg Oncol 1992; 18:937–940.
14. Zempsky WT, Parkinson TM. Lidocaine iontophoresis before shave biopsy. Dermatol Surg 2003; 29:627–630.
15. Nunez M, Miralles ES, Boixeda P. Iontophoresis for anesthesia during pulsed dye laser treatment of port wine stains. Pediatr Dermatol 1997; 14:397–340.
16. Kennard CD, Whitaker DC. Iontophoresis of lidocaine for anesthesia during pulsed dye laser treatment of port-wine stains. J Dermatol Surg Oncol 1992; 18:287–294.
17. Bezzant JL, Stephen RL, Petelenz TJ, et al. Painless cauterization of spider veins with the use of iontophoretic local anesthesia. J Am Acad Dermatol 1988; 19:869–875.
18. Decou JM, Abrams RS, Hammond JH, et al. Iontophoresis: a needle free, electrical system of local anesthesia delivery for pediatric surgical office procedures. J Pediatr Surg 1999; 34:946–949.
19. Squire SJ, Kirchoff KT, Hissong K. Comparing two methods of topical anesthesia used before intravenous cannulation in pediatric patients. J Pediatr Health Care 2000; 14:68–72.
20. Galankin JL, Rose JB, Harris K, et al. Lidocaine iontophoresis versus eutectic mixture of local anesthetics for IV placement in children. Anesth Analg 2002; 94:1484–1488.
21. Moppett IK, Szypula K, Yeoman PM. Comparison of EMLA and lidocaine iontophoresis for cannulation analgesia. Eur J Anesthesiol 2004; 21:210–213.
22. Miller KA, Balakrishnan G, Eichbauer G, et al. 1% lidocaine injection, EMLA cream or "numby stuff" for topical analgesia associated with peripheral intravenous cannulation. Am Anesth Nurs Assoc J 2001; 69:185–187.
23. Ashburn MA. The iontophoresis of lidocaine with epinephrine: an evaluation of depth and duration of skin anesthesia flowing short drug delivery times. Anesthesiology 1994; 81:A391.
24. Bjerring D, Arendt-Nielson L. Depth and duration of skin analgesia to needle insertion after topical application with EMLA cream. Br J Anaesth 1990; 64:173–177.
25. Ashburn M, Love G, Gaylord B, et al. Iontophoretic administration of 2% lidocaine HCL and 1:100,000 epinephrine in man. Clin J Pain 1997; 13:1322–1326.
26. Kearns GL, Heacook J, Daly SJ, et al. Percutaneous lidocaine administration via a new iontophoresis system in children: tolerability and absence of systemic bioavailability. Pediatrics 2003; 112:578–582.
27. Lesions and shocks during iontophoresis. Health Devices 1997; 23:123–125.
28. Rattenbury JM, Worthy E. Is the sweat test safe? Some instances of burns received during pilocarpine iontophoresis. Ann Clin Biochem 1996; 33:456–458.

9

Use of Nitrous Oxide in Hair Transplantation Surgery

Neil S. Sadick

Department of Dermatology, Joan and Sanford I. Weill Medical College and Weill Cornell Graduate School of Medical Sciences, Cornell University, New York, New York, U.S.A.

HISTORY

"Nitrous air" (a mixture of nitric oxide, nitrogen dioxide, and nitrous oxide) was first described by James Mayou, a 17th-century medical practitioner from Bath. The actual discovery of nitrous oxide is attributed to Joseph Priestly in 1772. Since its early use, nitrous oxide has passed through periods of greater and lesser popularity. However, its use for minor surgical procedures as a sole anesthetic agent as well as an adjunct to more potent inhalation agents continues to the present time.

PHARMACOKINETICS AND METABOLISM

Nitrous oxide (N_2O, dinitrogen monoxide) is a colorless gas with a slightly sweet odor. It stimulates the β-endorphin system, resulting in its euphoric and analgesic properties (1). In addition, nitrous oxide may also affect spinal interneurons directly, causing the release of enkephalins, which by inhibition of substance P may alter pain perception transmission via the spinothalamic route. It is marketed as a compressed liquid in equilibrium with its gaseous phase. As a result, the pressure in the tank remains nearly constant because liquid nitrous oxide returns to the gaseous phase as it is released from the cylinder. Although nonflammable, nitrous oxide supports combustion as actively as oxygen.

Recent studies have demonstrated region-dependent effects of N_2O on dopamine and/or norepinephrine concentrations or turnover in the brain (2,3) have provided further evidence for the involvement of dopamine and/or norepinephrine in transducing some of N_2O's effect in the central nervous system. Although the underlying mechanisms are unclear, several studies have suggested that N_2O releases opioid peptides in the central nervous system (4,5). In addition, there is much evidence that N_2O produces similar physiologic effects as opioids (6).

Results from recent studies have led to the hypothesis that N_2O-induced opioid peptides released in the periaqueductal gray area of the midbrain stimulate descending noradrenergic neuronal pathways that modulate nociceptive processing through the release of norepinephrine acting at Q2 adrenoceptors in the dorsal horn of the spinal cord (7,8).

A healthy adult breathing 70% nitrous oxide will achieve 90% equilibration in about 15 minutes. It is the least soluble of the inhalation anesthetics and thus achieves rapid equilibration between the alveoli partial pressure and the brain tissue partial pressure. This provides a rapid induction over a two- to three-minute period.

During the first 15 minutes, approximately 10 L of nitrous oxide will be absorbed from the alveoli into the circulation. The specifics of nitrous oxide metabolized are not completely understood; however, it is known that there is no significant metabolism of nitrous oxide in the liver (9,10). Anaerobic bacteria in the human intestine appear to metabolize it through a reductive pathway (10). Toxic by-products such as peroxidized lipids are formed and can be absorbed from the intestines. There is no evidence that absorption of these by-products has any clinical significance.

The combined use of nitrous oxide with propofol may decrease the recovery time and reduce postoperative nausea and vomiting that may be associated with propofol alone in office-based surgery (11).

DELIVERY SYSTEMS

The greatest risk in the use of nitrous oxide is the potential for the delivery of a hypoxic mixture ($O_2 < 21\%$). This is simply avoided with the use of proper equipment. Three basic features that increase safety in this setting are: (1) a fail-safe system, (2) a flowmeter arrangement, and (3) proportioning systems (Fig. 1).

Nitrous oxide and oxygen tanks are connected to the delivery system by a flowmeter designed to prevent delivery of hypoxic mixtures (Fig. 2). These

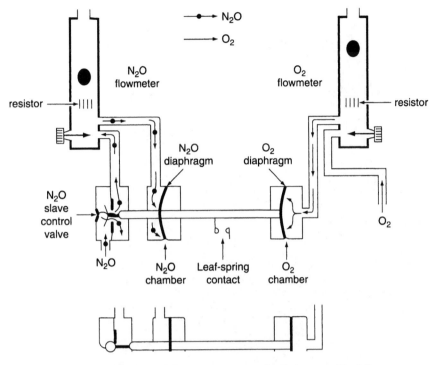

Figure 1 Schematic diagram of three component unit of nitrous oxide delivery system: (A) Fail-safe system, (B) Flowmeter, and (C) Proportioning system.

systems provide a fail-safe device that alarms automatically and turns off nitrous oxide flow should oxygen pressure be lost.

TECHNIQUES OF NITROUS OXIDE ADMINISTRATION

Nasal inhalers originally developed for dental procedures are the most suitable for use in office-based analgesia. The nasal inhaler should have a snug fit for the scavenging system to work appropriately. Three liter per minute of pure oxygen for the first three minutes should allow for denitrogenation; nitrous oxide can then be added to the mixture at 35% for another three minutes and will reduce pain associated with injection of local anesthetics. If analgesia is inadequate, nitrous oxide concentration can be safely increased to 66%. Total neurological recovery from nitrous oxide is usually fully achieved 10–20 minutes after its cessation.

INDICATIONS

Nitrous oxide has been used for hair transplantation procedures most commonly in conjunction with diazepam as a preanesthetic agent. The author has utilized this approach for the past two decades with great success and minimal side effect

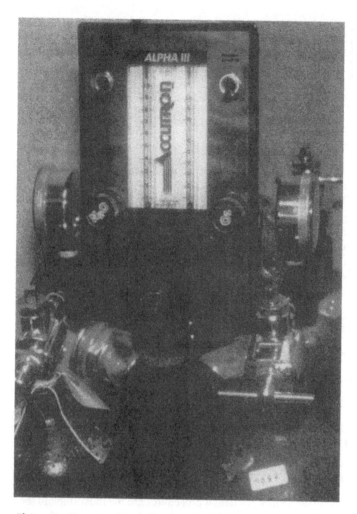

Figure 2 Nitrous oxide delivery system with separate nitrous oxide and oxygen tanks connected to the flowmeter delivery system.

profile. Shorter-acting benzodiazepines, e.g., midazolam, is preferred for shorter procedures.

A similar approach has been reported by Otley and Nguyen where a combination of oral diazepam and low to moderate concentrations of inhaled nitrous oxide produced good to excellent results in all patients. This approach was used in general dermatologic surgery as well as laser procedures in pediatrics (Table 1).

The author notes that training in conscious sedation as well basic and advanced cardiac life support should be a prerequisite for the practitioner (12).

Table 1 Characteristics of Patients and Sedation Outcome

Patient	Age (yr)	Sex	Condition/ procedure	Conscious sedation regimen	Quality of sedation	Complications
1	5	F	Nevus/ excision	Midazolam 12.5 mg by mouth (0.7 mg/kg); N_2O 30–50%; EMLA local anesthesia	Good	Nausea
2	16 (cognitive delay)	F	Metabolic disease/ biopsy	Diazepam 10 mg by mouth (0.3 mg/kg); N_2O 30–50%; EMLA	Excellent	None
3	17	M	Acute keloidosis/ excision	Lorazepam 2 mg by mouth; N_2O 35–50%; local anesthesia	Good	Nausea
4	5	F	Nevus/ excision	Midazolam 15 mg by mouth (0.8 mg/kg); N_2O 45% local anesthesia	Excellent	None
5	6	M	Nevus/ excision	Lorazepam 0.5 mg by mouth; N_2O 45%; local anesthesia	Excellent	None
6	11	M	Nevus/ excision	Lorazepam 0.5 mg by mouth; N_2O 35%; local anesthesia	Excellent	None
7	3	M	Pilomatricoma/ excision	Midazolam 12 mg by mouth (0.6 mg/kg); N_2O 45%; local anesthesia	Excellent	None
8	4	M	Wart/pulsed dye laser	Midazolam 12 mg by mouth (0.6 mg/kg); N_2O 45%; local anesthesia	Excellent	None
8	4	M	Wart/pulsed dye laser	Midazolam 12 mg by mouth (0.6 mg/kg); N_2O 45%; local anesthesia	Excellent	None

(*Continued*)

Table 1 Characteristics of Patients and Sedation Outcome (*Continued*)

Patient	Age (yr)	Sex	Condition/ procedure	Conscious sedation regimen	Quality of sedation	Complications
8	4	M	Wart/pulsed dye laser	Midazolam 12 mg by mouth (0.6 mg/kg); N$_2$O 45%; local anesthesia	Good	None
8	4	M	Wart/pulsed dye laser, curettage	Midazolam 12 mg by mouth (0.6 mg/kg); N$_2$O 45%; local anesthesia	Fair to poor	None

Abbreviations: EMLA, EMLA anesthetic cream (lidocaine 2.5% and prilocaine 2.5%); N$_2$O, nitrous oxide.

SIDE EFFECTS

Nitrous oxide is the most commonly used inhalation agent and is considered to have the highest margin of safety of all drugs currently in use for conscious sedation. It has a minimal depressive effect on the respiratory and cardiovascular systems (13,14). However, because of its poor solubility in blood, nitrous oxide rapidly exits the circulation into the alveoli with cessation of administration. This rapid diffusion of nitrous oxide dilutes alveolar oxygen concentration, producing diffusion hypoxia, which may last from one to two minutes. Hypoxia can be avoided by administering 100% oxygen for three to five minutes after nitrous oxide administration has been discontinued.

The effect of nitrous oxide on other organ systems varies widely. Nitrous oxide dilates cerebral blood vessels, thus increasing cerebral blood flow and intracranial pressure. The liver, kidney, and gastrointestinal tract show no marked effects. Fifteen percent of patients may suffer from nausea and vomiting postoperatively (14), which may be accompanied by transient light-headedness. Patients are advised to be either nil per os (NPO), that is, without oral foods or fluids or have only light meals prior to the administration of nitrous oxide.

Recently, reports of decreased fertility and an increased incidence of spontaneous miscarriage have been reported in medical personnel with chronic exposure to nitrous oxide (15–18). Sympathomimetic action of N$_2$O, i.e., α_1-adrenergic stimulation has been shown to play a partial role in N$_2$O-induced teratogenicity (19). Evacuation systems may be helpful in minimizing the exposure of medical personnel to nitrous oxide.

Sadick et al. studied the side effects of nitrous oxide in 200 hair transplant patients. He evaluated comparative pain responses in 50 patients where nitrous oxide was delivered by the Accutron Alpha III system with an average of 7 L of

Table 2   Comparison of Valium and Dermajet Vs. Nitrous Oxide
Preanesthesia—50-Patient Series

Anesthesia preference	Number of patients	Percentage
Valium/dermajet (1% lidocaine)	3	6
N$_2$O lidocaine	47	94

Table 3   Side Effects Nitrous Oxide—200 Patient Series

Side effects	Number of patients	Percentage
Mood lability	36	18
Nausea	12	6
Dizziness	5	2.5
Meaningless/disjointed verbal expressions	4	2
Stopped nitrous oxide due to uneasy feeling	4	2
Syncope	1	0.5
Respiratory depression	0	0
Arrhythmia APC	1	0.5
Hepatotoxicity	0	0
Malignant hyperthermia	0	0

Table 4   Mood Changes Induced by Nitrous Oxide in 36 Patients

Mood changes	Number of patients	Percentage
Laughter	28	78
Dissociation from surroundings	15	42
Anxiety	5	14
Crying	1	3
Hysteria	1	3
Delusions	1	3

nitrous oxide and 4 L of oxygen. This was compared to previous transplantation sessions utilizing 10 mg p.o. valium and Dermajet administration of 1% lidocaine (19) before lidocaine/epinephrine infiltration. Ninety-four percent of patients preferred nitrous oxide administration to valium/dermajet in terms of pain level during anesthetic infiltration of lidocaine/epinephrine (Table 2).

The most common side effect noted in the study was mood lability (Table 3) with laughter and dissociation from surroundings being the most common finding (Table 4). Feelings of uneasiness as well as syncope and atrial premature contractions may be related in part to anxiety and hyperventilation. Feelings of uneasiness, anxiety, syncope, and partial premature contractions as well as ventricular premature contractions have also been reported in hair transplantation patients receiving other preanesthetic and anesthetic agents (20,21). Crying, mild hysteria, and mild delusional states are extremely transient and can be intervened by lowering or discontinuing nitrous oxide administration (Table 4).

Nitrous oxide must be used with caution in patients with severe methylene tetrahydrofolate reductase (MTHFR) deficiency. Acute neurological deterioration was recently described in a pediatric patient with an MTHFR deficiency, leading to decreased 5-methyl tetrahydrofolate synthesis secondary to inactivation of methionine synthase by nitrous oxide resulting in extreme deficiency of methionine in the brain with ultimately death (22).

A primary advantage of nitrous oxide versus other preanesthetic agents, such as diazepam, meperidine, and atropine (used to reduce syncopal episodes), is that the side effects are short lived. The mood lability and gastrointestinal side effects are short lived, with immediate restoration of cognitive function after discontinuing nitrous oxide.

MANAGEMENT OF COMPLICATIONS

Recognition of early symptoms of an adverse reaction to nitrous oxide is of importance to prevent more serious complications. Mood lability, nausea, dizziness, and disjointed behavior should be managed by reducing nitrous oxide concentration in oxygen. If persistence of these symptoms continues, nitrous oxide should be completely discontinued and an alternate method of preanesthesia is instituted.

Syncopal episodes are managed by discontinuation of nitrous oxide, administration of 100% oxygen, and placing the patient in the head down position. Nausea and vomiting are usually self-limited with discontinuation of drug. Administration of 100% oxygen and treatment of hypoglycemia may be helpful in rapidly alleviating these symptoms.

Severe cardiorespiratory depression, arrhythmia, and malignant hyperthermia are serious but rare complications of nitrous oxide administration; it is prudent to have complete cardiovascular support equipment as well as competent personnel to manage such emergencies.

Procedures that require large large volumes of regional anesthetics in highly vascular areas, e.g., hair transplant, are better managed with nitrous oxide inhalation supplemented with benzodiazepine or analgesic.

CONCLUSION

Nitrous oxide is an excellent agent for dermatologic surgery. In hair transplantation surgery, it is very useful in reducing pain from local anesthetic infiltration. It has very few side effects that are transient if they do occur. The greatest advantage of nitrous oxide is its rapid onset of action and recovery, making it an ideal analgesic and anesthetic if combined with other drugs. When used as a single agent, total recovery occurs within minutes. Its safety and ease of administration cannot be overstated.

REFERENCES

1. Cruichshank JC, Sykes SH. Office sedation. Adv Dermatol 1992; 7:291–314.
2. Murakawa M, Adochi T, Nakao S, et al. Activation of the cortical and medullary dopanergic systems by nitrous oxide in rat: a possible neurochemical basis for psychotropic effects and post-anesthetic nausea and vomiting. Anesth Analg 1994; 78:376–381.
3. Karuria R, Kugel G, Engelking LR, et al. Alterations in catecholamine turnover in specific regions of the rat brain following acute exposure to nitrous oxide. Brain Res Bull 1998; 45:557–561.
4. Quack RM, Kouchick FJ, Tseng L. Influence of nitrous oxide upon region brain levels of methionine-enkephalin-like immunoreactivity in rats. Brain Res Bull 1986; 16:321–323.
5. Zuniga JR, Joseph SA, Knigge KM. The effects of nitrous oxide on the central endogenous pro-opiomelanocortin system in the rat. Brain Res 1987; 420:57–65.
6. Gillman MA, Lichtigfeld FJ. Pharmacology of psychotropic analgesic nitrous oxide—a multipotent opoid agonist. Int J Neurosci 1994; 76:5–12.
7. Maze M, Fujinaga M. Recent advances in understanding the actions and toxicity of nitrous oxide. Anesthesia 2000; 55:311–314.
8. Zhang C, Davies F, Guo TZ, et al. The analgesic action of nitrous oxide is dependent on the release of norepinephrine in the dorsal horn of the spinal cord. Anesthesiology 1999; 91:1401–1407.
9. Eger EL II. Cardiovascular effects of nitrous oxide. In: Eisele J, Jown N, eds. Nitrous Oxide/N_2O. New York: Elsevier, 1985:124–132.
10. Lampe GH, Wauk LZ, Whittendale D. Nitrous oxide does not impair hepatic function in young or old surgical patients. Anesth Analg 1990; 71:606–609.
11. Tang S, Lhen L, White P, et al. Use of propofol for office based anesthesia: effect of nitrous oxide on recovery profile. J Clin Anesth 1999; 11:226–230.
12. Otley CC, Nguyen TH. Conscious sedation of pediatric patients with combination of oral benzodiazepine and inhaled nitrous oxide. Dermatol Surg 2000; 26:1041–1044.
13. Griffin G, Campbell U, Jones R. Nitrous oxide—oxygen sedation for minor surgery. JAMA 1981; 245:2411–2413.
14. Gilman AG, Goodman LS, Trall TW, et al. General anesthetics. In: Price HL, Dripps RD, eds. The Pharmacological Basis of Therapeutics. Vol 6. New York: Macmillan, 1985:71–73.
15. Rowland AS, Weinberg CR, Baird DD, et al. Reduced fertility among women employed as dental assistants exposed to high levels of nitrous oxide. N Engl J Med 1992; 327:993–997.
16. Davis AG, Moir OP. Anesthesia during pregnancy. Clin Anaesth 1986; 4:233–246.
17. Crawford J, Lewis M. Nitrous oxide in early human pregnancy. Anesthesiology 1985; 41:900.
18. Aldridge LM, Tunstall ME. Nitrous oxide and the fetus: a review and the results of a retrospective study of 175 cases of anesthesia for insertion of Shroder sutures. Br J Anaesth 1986; 58(3):1348.
19. Fujinaga M, Baden JM, Suto A, et al. Preventative effects of phenoxybenzamine on nitrous oxide induced reproductive toxicity in Sprague-Dawley rats. Teratology 1991; 43:151–157.

20. Stegman SJ, Tromovitch TA, Glogau RG. In: Stegman SJ, Tromovitch TA, eds. Cosmetic Dermatologic Surgery. Chicago: Buck Medical Publisher, 1990; 93:77–120.
21. Alt TH. Hair transplantation and scalp reduction. In: Coleman III WP, Hanke CW, Alt TH, et al., eds. Cosmetic Surgery of the Skin. Philadelphia, PA: B.C. Decker, 1991:103–146.
22. Erbe RW, Solis RJ. Severe methylene tetrahydrofolate reductase deficiency, methionine synthesize and nitrous oxide—A cautionary tale. N Engl J Med 2003; 349:5–6.
23. De Castro G, Mundeleer P. Anesthesia sans sommeil "neuroleptanalgesie". Acta Chir Belg 1959; 58:689–693.
24. Kanmura V, Sakai J, Yashinaka H, et al. Causes of nitrous oxide contamination in operating rooms. Anesthesiology 1999; 90:693–696.
25. Lewis LA. Methoxyflurane analgesia for office surgery. J Dermatol Surg Oncol 1984; 10:85–86.
26. Norwood OT, Shiell RC. Anesthesia. In: Fox B, ed. Hair Transplant Surgery. Springfield, IL: Charles C. Thomas, 1990:245–265.
27. Sadick NS, Militana CJ. Use of nitrous oxide in hair transplantation surgery. J Dermatol Surg Oncol 1994; 20:186–190.

10

Moderate Sedation in Dermatologic Surgery

Omar Torres

*Cosmetic Surgery and Dermatology, PLLC,
St. Luke's-Roosevelt Medical Center, Department of
Dermatology, Columbia University, New York,
New York, U.S.A.*

Dwight Scarborough

*Cosmetic Surgery Center, Ohio State University,
Dublin, Ohio, U.S.A.*

Emil Bisaccia

*Department of Dermatology, Columbia
University, New York, New York, U.S.A.*

INTRODUCTION

As the range of acceptable ambulatory surgical patients and interventions continues to expand and the demand for cosmetic surgical procedures increases, it is of utmost importance that dermasurgeons possess a thorough knowledge of mild to moderate sedation and analgesia.

Moderate sedation/analgesia, formerly known as conscious sedation, is defined by the American Society of Anesthesiologist as a drug-induced depression of consciousness during which patients respond purposefully to verbal commands, either alone or accompanied by light tactile stimulation. In this state of mind, no interventions are required to maintain a patent airway, spontaneous ventilation is

Table 1 American Society of Anesthesiologists' Definitions of Levels of Sedation and Anesthesia

		Description
Level 1	Minimal sedation (anxiolysis)	A drug-induced state during which patients respond normally to verbal commands. Although cognitive function and coordination may be impaired, ventilatory and cardiovascular functions are unaffected
Level 2	Moderate sedation/ analgesia (conscious sedation)	A drug-induced depression of consciousness during which patients respond purposefully to verbal command, either alone or accompanied by light tactile stimulation. No interventions are required to maintain a patent airway, and spontaneous ventilation is adequate. Cardiovascular function is usually maintained
Level 3	Deep sedation/analgesia	A drug-induced depression of consciousness during which patients cannot be easily aroused but respond purposefully following repeated or painful stimulation. The ability to maintain independent ventilatory function may be impaired. Patients may require assistance in maintaining a patent airway, and spontaneous ventilation may be inadequate. Cardiovascular function is usually maintained
Level 4	Anesthesia	Consists of general anesthesia and spinal or major regional anesthesia. General anesthesia is a drug-induced loss of consciousness during which patients are not arousable, even by painful stimulation. The ability to maintain independent assistance in maintaining a patent airway and positive pressure ventilation may be required because of depressed spontaneous ventilation or drug-induced depression of neuromuscular function. Cardiovascular function may be impaired

adequate, and cardiovascular functions are unaffected. Table 1 summarizes the American Society of Anesthesiologist levels of sedation and anesthesia.

Local anesthesia may appear to be daunting to patients without sedation. Painful surgical procedures coupled with the inability to move for extended periods of time and the oftentimes negative emotional effects of visiting an operating room are often factors that merit the need for intravenous (IV) sedation. To date, no ideal anesthetic agent has been identified; instead, an array of drugs is used in order to accomplish a successful level of sedation.

Prior to administering IV sedation, the patient must undergo a comprehensive preoperative evaluation, obtain clearance from the primary care physician, and finally, refrain from consuming any food so that in the event of loss of airway reflexes, if deep sedation occurs, the risk of aspiration pneumonia is minimized.

PREREQUISITES FOR MODERATE SEDATION

A medical facility with outpatient surgery services and amenities should comply with the standards set forth by the Committee on Guidelines of Care of the American Academy of Dermatology, among others (1). These standards are intended to promote and ensure patient safety and facilitate the administration of anesthetics and lifesaving care.

First, the staff should be prepared and trained to resolve unexpected complications; surgeons, key medical personnel and anesthesiologists/CRNAs are required to obtain an Advanced Cardiac Life Support (ACLS) certification, and all nurses must have completed the basic life support (BLS) accreditation (2,3).

Moreover, the programmatic elements in a medical office where outpatient surgery is performed should be organized in a manner that enhances patient care and allows for close monitoring in the operating room as well as in the recovery room. At all times, two registered nurses will be stationed in the recovery room and will have easy access to the operating room to alert the staff in case of an emergency. Also, a telephone with a paging system is to be installed directly outside of the operating room for direct assistance. In the instance of an emergency where the patient must be admitted to a hospital, transportation agreements should be arranged beforehand (4–7).

Offices that administer IV sedation should be equipped with either wall source oxygen or portable oxygen tanks, portable or nonportable suction sources, emergency cardiac medications (Table 2), nasal oxygen cannulas, masks and ambubag, oral and nasal airways, endotracheal tubes and stylet, at least two

Table 2 Suggested Emergency Drugs

Oxygen	Lidocaine (cardiac, lidocaine, local infiltration)
Glucose (50%)	Naloxone hydrochloride
Atropine	Diphenhydramine hydrochloride
Epinephrine(1:1000, 1:10,000)	Hydrocortisone
Phenylephrine	Methylprednisolone
Dopamine	Succinycholine
Diazepam	Aminophylline
Isoproternol	Racemic epinephrine
Calcium chloride or calcium gluconate	Albuteron by inhalation
Sodium bicarbonate	Ammonia spirits

laryngoscopes, continuous pulse oximeter, continuous electrocardiograph, blood pressure monitor, IV access, antagonist medications, and protocols to obtain additional help.

Those in charge of the administering medication for anesthesia should possess formal training in clinical pharmacology and be legally authorized to supply anesthesia (8,9). The individual who administers anesthesia, such as an anesthesiologist or a certified registered nurse anesthetist (CRNA), is responsible for monitoring the patient under moderate sedation.

The CRNA, or trained anesthetist, is a key individual when it comes to monitoring the administration of anesthesia; otherwise, the surgeon could risk compromising the safety of the patient by concentrating too much of his or her efforts in keeping control over the administration of anesthetics. In any case, the surgeon must be knowledgeable of the agents used in anesthesia as well as understand physiologic monitoring and airway management, so as to take appropriate actions in case of complications.

PREOPERATIVE EVALUATION

In performing surgical procedures, the patient has to be informed of the risks and limitations of the procedure itself and the alternatives to moderate sedation. In cases where a surgical cosmetic procedure is involved, the patient must be made aware of the fact that postoperative results conform to realistic expectations. Prior to surgery, written preoperative instructions are to be given to the patient (Fig. 1).

For all surgical patients receiving presedation, the instructions listed below should be strictly followed regarding certain medications that should be taken upon rising, with just enough water to swallow the medication.

Intravenous sedation (similar to "twilight sleep") will be given by our anesthetist to eliminate any potential discomfort during the procedure. Discuss this with the doctor prior to surgery, and please be aware that it will necessitate having your doctor sign our medical clearance letter and arranging for you to have an ECG and chest x-ray.

If you routinely take specific medicines daily, on the day of your surgery you should plan to take:

Hypertension (high blood pressure) medications	Angina (heart-chest pain) medications
Asthma medications	Convulsion-prevention medications
Cardiac dysrhythmias (irregular heartbeat) medication	Parkinson's medications
Any other heart medication that you take on a regular basis	Discuss with the doctor any diabetic medications

---

Figure 1 (*Continued*)

DO NOT TAKE :

Anticoagulants (blood-thinners or any form of aspirin). If you take an anticoagulant on a regular basis, please check with your doctor. It may be necessary to change your medication to a shorter-acting type several days in advance of your surgery.

Despite the many benefits, some vitamins and herbal remedies can have detrimental effects on a person undergoing surgery.

Herbal and other Remedies Possible Complications

Aspirin	Increases bleeding and bruising.
Ibuprofen	Increases bleeding and bruising
Nonsteroidal anti-inflammatory drugs (NSAIDS)	Increases bleeding and bruising
Selenium, chromium, vitamin E	Antiplatelet activity and induces bleeding.
Ginger, garlic, cayenne and bilberry	Antiplatelet activity and induces bleeding.
Ginkgo biloba	Powerful anticoagulant and induces bleeding
Aloe	Topical can cause dermatitis.
Vitamin A	Liver toxicity in high amounts.
St. John's wort, yohimbine, and licorice root	May intensify effects and potency of anesthesia
Ginseng and Ma-huang extract (6% ephedrine)	May induce high blood pressure and rapid heart rate.

MODERATE SEDATION—PREOPERATIVE INSTRUCTIONS

Except for the sips of clear liquids needed to take any of the above medications, it is very important that each patient not eat solid food or drink milk for eight (8) hours prior to the scheduled surgery.

No food or drink after midnight if twilight sleep or presedation is to be administered. Please refer to the following diet guidelines:

1. No solid food or milk after midnight on the day of surgery.
2. Unlimited clear liquid from the list below may be taken up to 3 hours before the scheduled time of surgery. After this time, only oral medications may be taken. Oral medication should be taken with no more than 1 ounce of water up to 1 hour before surgery.

ONLY CLEAR LIQUIDS ARE ACCEPTABLE

Water, black coffee or tea (no milk, cream, or non-diary creamer), apple juice (clear), club soda, ginger ale, Seven-Up, Cola.

If there are any questions as to whether a medication should be taken on the day of your surgery, please contact us at ( ) _____

These instructions concern only medicines you take at home before coming to our office. Your anesthetic and any medications that you will receive here will be discussed with you on your surgery day.

Figure 1 Moderate sedation—preoperative instructions.

Table 3 American Society of Anesthesiologists' Physical Status
Classification System

Classification	Description
I	A normal healthy individual
II	A patient with mild to moderate systemic disease
III	A patient with severe systemic disease that is not incapacitation
IV	A patient with incapacitating systemic disease that is a constant threat to life
V	A moribund patient who is not expected to survive 24 hr without operation

The American Society of Anesthesiologists' Physical Status Classification System categorizes patients in types I, II, III, IV, and V (Table 3) (10). Type I and II patients are the most appropriate candidates for outpatient moderate sedation.

Prior to sedation, the patient will have obtained medical clearance by the primary care physician (Fig. 2) (11). To obtain medical clearance, the patient must undergo a preliminary physical exam. In addition, an evaluation of the cardiopulmonary system, reactions to previous sedative or analgesics, and use of medications, especially those that could interact with the sedatives or preclude clotting, must be evaluated (11).

PERIOPERATIVE MONITORING

In cases where patients receive moderate sedation, they are monitored following the Joint Commission on Accreditation of Healthcare Organizations (JCAHO) guidelines (12,13). JCAHO defines patient monitoring as follows.

Appropriate equipment for care and resuscitations is available for the continuous monitoring of the vital signs. This includes heart rate, respiratory rates, and oxygenation using a transcutaneous pulse oximeter. Blood pressure should be measured at regular intervals. All patients, especially those with a history of significant cardiovascular disease or dysrythmias, should be monitored with electrocardiography (12,13).

Pulse oximeters measure the saturation of oxygen in arteries (Sao_2), which are accurate in the 70–100% range (14), and are quantified as oxygen saturation pulse (Spo_2). Arrhythmias, cardiac arrest, hypovolemia, hypothermia, vaso-constriction, anemia, injection of dyes, and dyshemoglobin are internal factors that can alter the readings for the oxygen saturation pulse (Spo_2) (14). Several external factors can affect the Spo_2 reading as well, such as an inflated blood pressure cuff, nail polish or synthetic nails, ambient light, electrocautery, and

Date: _____

RE: _____

Dear Doctor :

I have recently seen the above named patient who is considering a cosmetic surgical procedure.

Prior to undergoing this procedure, I have asked him/her to see you to obtain a complete physical examination, including a chest x-ray and EKG. The following levels will be obtained at our office two weeks prior to surgery.

- SMAC   - Bleeding Time
- CBC with differential   - T-4
- PT   - Urinalysis
- PTT   - HIV screening
- Platelets- Serum Pregnancy Test
- Fibrinogen Level (If female of childbearing age)
- Hepatitis Bag

Please indicate by letter or use of this form, whether or not you feel this patient's current physical condition makes them a reasonable candidate for this procedure, along with forwarding a copy of all test results. If you have any questions, please don't hesitate to contact me.

Very Truly Yours,

PHYSICIAN STATEMENT:

I have determined by history and physical examination that this patient is and acceptable candidate for outpatient surgery, provided the above lab tests are within normal limits.

_____   _____   _____
       Signature   Printed Name   Date

Figure 2 Sample of a medical clearance letter to be filled out by primary physician.

Table 4 Ramsey Sedation Scale

Levels	Characteristics
I	Anxious, agitated, restless
II	Cooperative, oriented, or tranquil
III	Drowsy, but responding to commands
IV	Asleep but exhibiting a brisk response to stimuli
V	Asleep and exhibiting a sluggish response to stimuli
VI	Asleep with no response to stimuli

movement of the fingers. Cardiac performance should be monitored through an electrocardiogram since Spo$_2$ does not correlate with myocardium oxygenation in every instance (14).

When oxygen saturation levels drop below 90%, it is necessary to revert this via corrective measures (i.e., jaw thrust maneuver and oral secretion suctioning). Table 4 describes the Ramsay scale (15), which quantifies drug-induced sedation according to the patients' responsiveness.

An additional avenue to closely monitor the levels of sedation consists of the electroencephalogram (EEG). The EEG-BIS index is a computerized analysis that identifies pain impulses in the brain. The EEG-BIS index simplifies EEG interpretations and is a useful resource to monitor the administration of sedative drugs (16). However, for moderate sedation purposes, the EEG-BIS index is helpful, but not necessary. In moderate sedation, by titrating to effect, enough sedation and analgesia is achieved while simultaneously allowing the patient to move if any discomfort is experienced.

INTRAVENOUS ANESTHETIC DRUGS

An ideal sedative-hypnotic should induce analgesia, sedation, and amnesia, as well as calm the patient and depress coughing, laryngospasm, and gagging, all the while allowing for the patient to remain cooperative. It should also create minimal or no depression of the cardiovascular, respiratory, and central nervous systems. Despite the fact that no drug has been found to contain all these properties, the best drug combination possible should be administered to ensure a safe and pleasant sedation. Our preferred moderate sedation protocol is outlined in Table 5.

Benzodiazepines

Benzodiazepines are the most widely used anxiolytic drugs and preferred preoperative sedative in adults (17). Their mechanism of action is mediated by binding to a specific receptor, which is adjacent to the γ-aminobutyric acid (GABA) receptor. The benzodiazepines enhance GABA affinity to its receptor

Table 5 Continuous Infusion Technique

1.	Intravenous line established (Ringer's lactate, normal saline, etc.)
2.	Midazolam 0.05 to 0.75 mg/kg (slow titration)
3.	Fentanyl 1 to 2 μg/kg (for select cases only)
4.	Initiate sedation slowly with a continuous infusion technique to achieve the desired level of conscious sedation as measured by the Ramsey scale
5.	Begin propofol administration (25 to 50 μg/kg/min)
6.	Infusion rate may be increased at 5 μg/kg/min
7.	Look for signs of clinical end point of conscious sedation (nystagmus, slurred speech) at dosage ranges of 0.5 to 2 mg/kg/min. Slowly establish dosage and rate of administration. Total dosage may need to be adjusted accordingly to the patient's preprocedure status, age, presence of disease, and desired level of sedation

allowing a greater entry of chloride into the cell, inhibiting neuronal firing. Benzodiazepines—useful drugs for ambulatory surgery—produce sedation, hypnosis, anxiolysis, and amnesia. They are muscle relaxant and, in some instances, anticonvulsants.

Midazolam is the most commonly used benzodiazepine for preprocedure and for intraprocedure sedation, anxiolysis, and amnesia because of its safe pharmacokinetics (rapid onset and short duration of action) (18). Midazolam mildly affects the cardiovascular and respiratory system. When compared with other benzodiazepines, midazolam has obvious advantages due to its solubility in water, short latency, short elimination half-life, and higher rate of clearance (18). The recommended midazolam dose of 0.1 to 0.15 mg/kg IV in divided doses is adequate for moderate sedation in a healthy individual. Caution should be taken with the higher end of this dosing range since it can cause significant respiratory depression especially in the elderly (19).

Barbiturates

The barbiturates are derivatives of barbituric acid and have been used since the beginning of the 20th century. Once the mainstay of treatment for sedation and anesthesia, barbiturates have been replaced by benzodiazepines and other newer drugs that do not cause physical dependence, induce tolerance, or are associated with severe withdrawal symptoms. Barbiturates are not analgesic and do require some type of supplementary analgesia. In addition, they depress the cardiovascular and respiratory systems.

Thiopental (2.5–4.5 mg/kg), an ultra-short-acting barbiturate (duration of action around 20 minutes), is still the most widely used IV general anesthesia inductor agent (20). Thiopental can impair fine motor movements for several hours after surgery. Methohexital has a shorter awakening time when compared to thiopental but requires a 6- to 8-hour recovery period. Methohexital compared favorably with propofol for induction of procedures lasting more than two hours (21).

Secobarbital and pentobarbital, which are short-acting barbiturates, with a 3- to 5-hour average duration of action, are used as preoperative sedatives. Postoperatively, they have shown to cause less nausea and vomiting than opioids.

To date, there is no specific pharmacologic antagonist to treat barbiturate overdose; therefore, maintaining an airway, support ventilation, and circulation are the proper symptomatic treatments.

Ketamine

As opposed to other anesthetic induction agents, ketamine induces "dissociative" anesthesia where the patient appears to be awake but is in a state of profound analgesia and amnesia; it works as a noncompetitive antagonist of the *N*-methyl-D-aspartate (NMDA) glutamate receptor. Antimuscarinic and anticholinergic properties appear to be clinically relevant as well (22). Studies have shown that the administration of ketamine before painful stimulus resulted in an average reduction of 40–60% in the amount of opioids requirements after surgery (23).

At small doses (0.1–0.5 mg/kg IV or 2–4 mg/kg IM), ketamine induces good analgesia, which can be used to supplement local anesthesia in cosmetic surgical procedures. Ketamine has a relatively short distribution and short elimination half-lives (around 2–3 hours); it stimulates the heart and increases the blood pressure, heart rate, and cardiac output. It is a bronchodilator causing minimal depression of the respiratory system, but stimulates salivary and tracheobronchial secretions, and concurrent administration of an anticholinergic, such as glycopyrrolate, is recommended (24). Because of postoperative hallucinations, ketamine is used in small doses with other medications, mostly benzodiazepines.

Pediatric patients have fewer adverse emergence reactions than adults and it can be administered orally, which makes ketamine a well-considered choice for sedation for infants.

Propofol

Propofol is a diisopropylphenol, a new category of IV sedative hypnotics. It is short-acting and has a rapid onset of action and a clearance, which is 10 times that of thiopental (25). Propofol is a potent respiratory depressant; therefore, oxygen should be supplemented. Because of its rapid induction and emergence, propofol is suited for outpatient cosmetic procedures. It compares favorably with midazolam in that it allows for a more rapid recovery of cognitive functions and less postoperative sedation, drowsiness, confusion, and amnesia. Side effects include pain on injection, involuntary movement, hypotension, excitatory phenomena, and depressed myocardial contractility (26). Venous pain from propofol injection at the hands has been shown to be reduced with lidocaine (40 mg IV) immediately before the infusion of propofol (27).

In 2059 office-based plastic surgery procedures reported by Friedberg, the combination of 2-mg midazolam and propofol infusion until sleep followed by the administration of 50 mg of ketamine prior to the application of local anesthesia and further continuation with a propofol drip resulted in very safe sedation and analgesia with fast postoperative recovery (28). Since propofol use is associated with a low incidence of postoperative nausea and vomiting (PONV), less usage of antiemetic drugs is necessary. Propofol is an aqueous solution devoid of preservatives and is, hence, a potential vector of infections. Therefore, the manufacturer's recommendations should be followed closely (29).

ANALGESICS

Opioids

Because of their analgesic properties, opioids are commonly used during surgery and in postsurgical pain control management. Opioids can induce sedation, analgesia, muscle rigidity, and euphoria (30). Fentanyl (1–3 µg/kg), alfentanil (1–20 µg/kg), and sufentanil (0.1–0.3 µg/kg) produce a strong, short-lasting analgesia when administered via IV boluses.

Fentanyl is a highly potent opioid, which has a rapid onset and short duration of action of approximately 15 to 30 minutes. Although fentanyl is less likely to induce nausea than other opioids, it could activate a cholinergic action resulting in bradycardia (30).

ANTAGONISTS

Flumazenil

Flumazenil is a high-affinity competitive antagonist at the benzodiazepine receptor that reverses the sedation of a patient who remains depressed after administration of a benzodiazepine. Flumazenil is cleared relatively fast and has a half-life of 0.7 to 1.3 hours (31). Monitoring should be done when reversing the effects of a long-lasting benzodiazepine with a single dose of flumazenil due to potential resedation. A dose of 0.1 to 0.2 mg IV administered every minute up to 3.0 mg has been proven to reverse the effects of diazepam, lorazepam, midazolam, and flunitrazepam (32).

Naloxone, Naltrexone, and Nalmefene

Nalxone, naltrexone, and nalmefene are opioid competitive antagonists used to reverse opioid-induced coma and respiratory depression. They displace opioid molecules bound to receptors κ, µ, and σ. In the spinal cord, κ receptor agonists have been shown to mediate analgesia. They have a much higher affinity to µ receptors, which may explain why they are able to reverse respiratory depression with only minimal reversal of analgesia. Naloxone can be administered at a dose of 0.2 to 0.4 mg IV at a rate of 0.2 mg every two minutes until reaching the desire clinical response (33). Because of its short half-life (0.5–1.5 hours), it should be administered continuously, at one- to two-hour intervals, to maintain the antagonistic effects (34).

Naltrexone is also a κ-, μ-, and σ-opioid receptor antagonist. As opposed to naloxone, it has a longer half-life (8–12 hours) and can be taken orally.

Nalmefene is another κ-, μ-, and σ-opioid receptor antagonist, which can be administered orally or parenterally. Its half-life has been reported to range from 3 to 10 hours depending on the dosage used (35).

ANTIEMETICS

Nausea can complicate the postoperative recovery time. In view of the fact that opioids are one of the leading causes of nausea, their administration should be minimized. Dehydration, pain, obesity, pregnancy, age, gender, phase of menstrual cycle, postural hypotension, increased gastric volume, type of anesthesia or analgesia used, and a history of motion sickness have been associated to a higher risk for PONV (36–39). Because of the low incidence of PONV after moderate sedation, the possible adverse effects of these agents, and steep costs associated with this drug, prophylactic use of antiemetics should not be used in every patient. In a high-risk patient for PONV, a single or a combination of medications can be used. A brief description of different classes of antiemetic agents is outlined below.

Butyrophenones

Droperidol at a dose of 0.005 to 0.07 mg/kg IV is an effective antiemetic agent because of its anti-dopamine properties. Higher doses are not recommended due to a potential increase in the postoperative sedation and other adverse effects, which can prolong the recovery time (40). Because of stringent FDA warning of droperidol association with sudden death, the drug has been removed from most hospital formularies in the United States.

Gastrokinetic Agents

Metoclopramide and domperidone are gastrokinetic agents. Metoclopramide (10 mg IV) has shown to reduce the incidence of nausea and vomiting when administered before induction of anesthesia (41).

Anticholinergics

Scopolamine, atropine, and glycopyrrolate are some of the anticholinergics used as antiemetics (42). Scopolamine patch has been shown to reduce PONV in high-risk patients if it is applied approximately 8 hours prior to surgery. Some of the side effects associated with anticholinergics are dry mouth, blurring of vision, tachycardia, and constipation.

Phenothiazines

Prochlorperazine and promethazine are useful in the treatment of PONV, especially when caused by previous administration of opioids. Both drugs come in a 25-mg suppository, and a normal dose for an adult is 25 mg every 12 hours. These neuroleptic drugs can cause hypotension and sedation, and other adverse extrapyramidal effects (43).

Serotonin Antagonists

Ondansetron is one of the most efficacious antiemetic drugs. It blocks 5-HT$_3$ receptors, both centrally and peripherally. It comes in an aqueous solution for IV or IM administration. It is also available in tablets, oral solution, and orally disintegrating tablets. All these presentations make ondansetron a versatile antiemetic drug that can be used prophylactically against PONV in high-risk patients or acutely in patients with ongoing symptoms. Headache and liver enzyme elevation are among its most common side effects (44–46).

INHALATION ANESTHESIA

Nitrous Oxide

Nitrous oxide (N$_2$O) produces anxiolysis and mild analgesic effects. N$_2$O and oxygen are usually given at an initial flow rate of 6 L/min each; after approximately 1 minute, the flow rates are reduced to 3 L/min for both gases (47). N$_2$O has a very low solubility in the blood; therefore, it produces a fast induction and recovery. Because of the risk of hypoxia, it is never to be given in concentrations above 80%.

Because of its safety and ability to be administered intranasally, it is preferred in the pediatric population. Studies have shown that N$_2$O and at least 30% oxygen prior to infiltration of local anesthesia reduce anxiety and pain (48). When used alone and at low concentrations, no monitoring is required, since the patient retains all reflexes.

By itself, it does not produce surgical anesthesia; thus, it is commonly used in conjunction with other anesthetics, usually a benzodiazepine. With this regimen, respiratory depression is the most likely complication; therefore, monitoring of the airways, ventilation, and oxygenation is of extreme importance.

Around 15% of patients will develop nausea and vomiting postoperatively. Nitrous oxide is flammable, and safety measures should be taken to avoid fire.

Alert, oriented, responds coherently to questioning

Hemodynamically stable when standing and sitting

Neurologically intact, ambulating with minimal assistance

Has voided postprocedure

Oral intake maintained

Discharged to a responsible third party

Figure 3   Patient discharge criteria.

POSTOPERATIVE RECOVERY

Patient response to command occurs within 3 to 7 minutes after discontinuing IV propofol administration. A prolonged recovery could be owed to a higher concentration in the dosage, the speed of infiltration, and the pharmacokinetic of the anesthetic itself.

Toward the end of the procedure, the amount of sedation administered is reduced due to the ongoing effects of the previously infiltrated local anesthetics. At this time, the patient gradually wakes up. Postoperative wound care stimulates the patient and signals the completion of the procedure. The patient can then ambulate with assistance to the postoperative recovery area (11,49).

In the recovery area, patients are monitored for at least 30 minutes, and vital signs are recorded every 5 to 10 minutes. If the patient shows signs of normal recuperation, vital signs can be checked every 15 minutes until he or she is ready for discharge. Discharge criteria and instructions are outlined in Figures 3 and 4. Next, the IV line is removed, and the patient is taken to the bathroom to void (11,49).

The patient is now ready for discharge under the care of an adult and should schedule postoperative follow-up appointments. Additionally, a series of postoperative written instructions and an emergency contact number are provided to the patient at the time of discharge.

SUMMARY

Moderate sedation is a suitable anesthetic option for outpatient surgery in the proper setting that will yield successful results when administered correctly; it maximizes physician efficiency and allows for the patient's rapid recovery with minimal side effects. However, it is important to note that the medical facility and the staff must meet specific criteria to ensure successful results; the office

---

For patients who have had : _____ Spinal epidural

_____ Local anesthesia with sedation

_____ Nerve block

_____ General anesthesia

_____ Conscious sedation

The medicine that was used to sedate you will be acting in you body for the next 24 hours. As a result, you might feel a little sleepy or dizzy when you get home. This feeling will slowly wear off.

- For the next 24 hours you should not:
- Drive a car; operate machinery or power tools, etc.
- Drink any alcoholic beverages, even beer
- Take any medication not prescribed by your physician
- Make any important decisions, such as to sign important papers.

You may eat anything, but it is better to start with liquids such as soft drinks (soda), then go on to soup and crackers and gradually work up to more solid foods. It is not uncommon to be a little nauseated after surgery.

We strongly suggest that a responsible adult be with you for the rest of the day and also during the night for your protection and safety. After 24 hours, you may resume your daily activities within the limits set by the surgeon.

You may experience a slight sore throat and/or some degree of muscle soreness after the anesthetic. This is not uncommon and should clear up quickly. It is due to breathing though you mouth while you were lightly sedated, not unlike snoring.

If you receive a nerve block, the anesthetized body part may not have the normal sensations that usually protect it from injury. Care must be taken to protect the anesthetized area until full sensation returns.

If any questions should arise, call the office immediately at ( )_____

Figure 4 Moderate sedation outpatient discharge instructions. *Source*: From Ref. 50.

will be designed and equipped to promote the safety of the patient, and the staff will possess the training and skills to provide appropriate care. In addition, proper patient selection and a thorough understanding of the medications used during the procedure as well as possible complications management are required.

Dermasurgeons whose practice involves performing invasive procedures will find moderate sedation an optimal anesthetic technique applicable for a vast array of procedures, with a proven track needed for safety in outpatient surgery.

REFERENCES

1. Committee on Guidelines of Care for Office Surgical Facilities, part I. J Am Acad Dermatol 1992; 5:763–765.
2. Chrisman BB. Planning and staffing an appropriate outpatient facility. J Dermatol Surg Oncol 1988; 7:708–711.
3. Penn JG, Baker JL. The office-based elective surgery center. Ann Plast Surg 1980; 2:94–99.
4. Elliot RA, Hoehn JG. The office surgical suite-the physical plant and equipment. Clin Plast Surg 1983; 10:269–272.
5. Fader DJ, Johnson TM. Medical issues and emergencies in the dermatologic office. J Am Acad Dermatol 1997; 36:1–16.
6. Gilbert DA, Adamson JE. Procedure manuals in office surgery. Clin Plast Surg 1980; 2:94–99.
7. Kanter MA. The prevention and management of medical problems during office surgery. Plast Reconstr Surg 1990; 85:1227–1368.
8. White PF. Ambulatory anesthesia—fast tracking concepts. Anesth Anal 1998; 103 (suppl 153–156).
9. Odom J. Tips for RN-administered conscious sedation. Todays Surg Nurs 1996; 18:22–25.
10. American Society of Anesthesiology: new classification of physical status. Anesthesiology 1963; 24:111.
11. Abeles G, Warmuth IP, Sequeira M, et al. The use of conscious sedation for outpatient dermatologic surgical procedures. Dermatol Surg 2000; 26:121–126.
12. Joint Commission on Accreditation for Health Care Organizations. Comprehensive accreditation manual for hospitals; the official handbook. Oak Brook Terrace, IL: Joint Commission on Accreditation of Heath Care Organizations, 2000.
13. New definitions: revised standards address the continuum of sedation and analgesia. Jt Comm Perspect 2000; 20:10–12.
14. Burns LS. Advances in pediatric anesthesia. Nurs Clin North Am 1986; 32:45–71.
15. Standard Policy for Conscious Sedation. Grant/Riverside Hospital, Ohio Health Systems. December 1, 1997.
16. Sa Rêgo MM, Watcha MF, White PF. Then changing role of monitored anesthesia care in the ambulatory setting. Anesth Analg 1997; 85:1020–1036.
17. White PF. Pharmacologic and clinical aspects of preoperative medication. Anesth Analg 1986; 65:693–694.
18. Khanderia U, Pandit SK. Use of midazolam hydrochloride in anesthesia. Clin Pharm 6:533–547, 1987.
19. Dundee JW, Haslett WH. The benzodiazepines: a review of their actions and uses relative to anesthetic practice. Br J Anaesth 1970; 42:217–234.
20. Avram MJ, Sanghvi R, Henthorn TK, et al. Determinants of thiopental induction dose requirements. Anesth Analg 1993; 76:10–17.

21. Sun R, Skrivanek G, Stool L, et al. Use of methohexital for induction of outpatient anesthesia: a cost-effective alternative to propofol? Anesth Analg 1997; 84:S29.
22. Coté CJ. Sedation for the pediatric patient. A review. Pediatr Clin North Am 1994; 41:31–50.
23. Fu ES, Miguel R, Scharf JE. Preemptive ketamine decreases postoperative narcotic requirements in patients undergoing abdominal surgery. Anesth Analg 1997; 84: 1086–1090.
24. Kohrs R, Durieux ME. Ketamine: teaching an old drug new tricks. Anesth Analg 1998; 87:1186–1193.
25. Smith I, White PF, Nathanson M, et al. Propofol: an update on its clinical use. Anesthesiology 1994; 81:1005.
26. Bryson HM, Fulton BR, Faulds D. Propofol an update of its use in anaesthesia and conscious sedation. Drugs 1995; 50:513–559.
27. Haugen RD, Vaghadia H, Waters T, et al. Thiopentone pretreatment for propofol injection pain in ambulatory patients. Can J Anaesth 1995; 42:1108.
28. Friedberg BL. Propofol ketamine anesthesia for cosmetic surgery in office suite. Int Anesthesiol Clin 2003; 41:39–50.
29. Lorenz IH, Kolbitsch C, Lass-Florl C, et al. Routine handling of propofol prevents contaminations as effectively as does strict adherence to the manufacturer's recommendations. Can J Anaesth 2002; 49:347–352.
30. Bailey PL, Egan TD, Stanley TH. Intravenous opioids anesthetics. In: Miller RD, ed. Anesthesia. 5th ed. Philadelphia: Churchill Livingstone, 2000:273–376.
31. Koltz U. Drug interactions and clinical pharmacokinetics of flumazenil. Eur J Anaesthesiol 1988; 2:103.
32. Whitwam JG, Amrein R. Pharmacology of flumazenil. Acta Anaesthesiol Scand Suppl 1995; 108:3.
33. Wood M. Opioid agonists and antagonists. In: Wood M, Wood AJJ, eds. Drugs and Anesthesia: Pharmacology for Anesthesiologists. Baltimore: Williams & Wilkins, 1990.
34. Alexander JI, Hill RG. Postoperative Pain Control. Boston: Blackwell Scientific, 1987.
35. Glass PSA, Jhaveri RM, Smith LR. Comparison of potency and duration of action of nalmefene and naloxone. Anesth Analg 1994; 78:536–541.
36. Lerman J. Surgical and patient factors involved in postoperative nausea and vomiting. Br J Anaesth 1992; 69: S24–S32.
37. Watch M, White P. Postoperative nausea and vomiting: its etiology, treatment, and prevention. Anesthesiology 1992; 77:162–184.
38. Cohen MM, Duncan PG, DeBoer DP, et al. The postoperative interview: assessing risk factors for nausea and vomiting. Anesth Analg 1994; 78:7–16.
39. Watcha MF, White PF. The postoperative nausea and vomiting: its etiology, treatment, and prevention. Anesthesiology 1992; 77:162.
40. Melnick B, Sawyer R, Karambelkar D, et al. Delayed side effects of droperidol after ambulatory general anesthesia. Anesth Analg 1989; 69:748.
41. Madej TH, Simpson KH. Comparison of the use of domperidone, droperidol and metoclopramide in the prevention of nausea and vomiting following gynaecological surgery in day cases. Br J Anaesth 1986; 58:879–883.
42. Bailey PL, Streisand JB, Pace NL, et al. Transdermal scopolamine reduces nausea and vomiting after outpatient laparoscopy. Anesthesiology 1990; 72:977–980.

43. Watcha MF, White PF. New antiemetic drugs. Int Anesthesiol Clin 1995; 33:1.
44. Bodner M, White PF. Antiemetic efficacy of ondansetron after outpatient laparo-scopy. Anesth Analg 1991; 73:250–254.
45. Scuderi P, Wetchler B, Sung YF, et al. Treatment of postoperative nausea and vomiting after outpatient surgery with the 5-HT3 antagonist ondansetron. Anesthe-siology 1993; 78:15–20.
46. Sung YF, Wetchler BV, Duncalf D, et al. A double-blind, placebo-controlled pilot study examining the effectiveness of intravenous ondansetron in the prevention of postoperative nausea and emesis. J Clin Anesth 1993; 5:22–29.
47. Goldman MP, Fitzpatrick RE. Anesthesia for cutaneous laser surgery. In: Goldman MP, Fitzpatrick RE, eds. Cutaneous Laser Surgery: The Art and Science of Selective Photodermolysis. Mosby: St. Louis, 1994:269–282.
48. Maloney JM, Coleman WP, Mora R. Analgesia induced by nitrous oxide and oxygen as an adjunct to local anesthesia in dermatologic surgery—results of clinical trials. J Dermatol Surg Oncol 1980; 6:939–943.
49. Scarborough DA, Bain-Herron J, Khan A, et al. Experience with more than 5000 cases in which monitored anesthesia care was used for liposuction surgery. Aesthetic Plast Surg 2004; 27:474–480.
50. Bisaccia E, Scarborough DA. Anesthesia. In: The Columbia Manual of Dermatologic Cosmetic Surgery. New York: McGraw-Hill, 2002.

Index